£25.99

Essential Radiological Anatomy for the MRCS

Essential Radiological Anatomy for the MRCS

Stuart Currie

Steven Kennish

and

Karen Flood

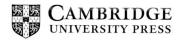

CAMBRIDGE
UNIVERSITY PRESS

CAMBRIDGE UNIVERSITY PRESS

Cambridge, New York, Melbourne, Madrid, Cape Town, Singapore, São Paulo, Delhi

Cambridge University Press
The Edinburgh Building, Cambridge CB2 8RU, UK

Published in the United States of America by Cambridge University Press, New York

www.cambridge.org
Information on this title: www.cambridge.org/9780521728089

First published 2009

Printed in the United Kingdom at the University Press, Cambridge

A catalogue record for this publication is available from the British Library

ISBN 978-0-521-72808-9 paperback

To our loving families

Contents

Preface

Nearly all surgical patients undergo some form of radiological imaging as part of their diagnostic work-up. It is often the role of the surgical trainee to clerk and examine the patient, and initiate emergent treatment and investigations in the acute setting. A basic understanding of the role of imaging and its demonstration of relevant anatomy is a fundamental prerequisite to the appropriate utilization of the radiological armamentarium.

Surgical trainees are not expected to interpret imaging to the point of issuing a report; this is the role of the radiologist. Sound knowledge of radiological anatomy can prove invaluable however in the initial reviewing of plain films, and give the surgeon a more informed opinion in the radiological multidisciplinary meeting.

Over recent years the Membership of the Royal College of Surgeons (MRCS) viva examination has increasingly made use of radiological imaging to facilitate the discussion of anatomy relevant to every day surgical practice. Indeed, the authors were questioned on sagittal magnetic resonance images of the brain, male and female pelvis and radiographs of the chest and abdomen.

For many, examinations are stressful. The last thing a candidate needs is to be faced with unfamiliar radiological images. This review of surgically relevant radiological imaging aims to prevent initial uncertainties, and should allow the candidate to rapidly progress to confidently discussing the anatomy and scoring valuable points.

This book aims to provide you with a number of key advantages before entering the exam. Firstly, you will become familiar with a range of images of differing modalities (plain film, fluoroscopy, computed tomography and magnetic resonance imaging). Secondly, different planes of imaging are utilized, so that you will not be fazed by an unusual coronal or sagittal view. You are also provided with 'favourite' anatomy viva questions and concise but detailed notes. Finally, the anatomical notes are correlated with surgical scenarios enabling you to read around potential topics for clinical discussion.

How to use this book

Prerequisites

By convention, radiological images are presented in a way that equates to you looking at the 'anatomical man' face to face. The patient's right is therefore found on the left-hand side of the image and vice versa, a so-called mirror image effect. This applies to cross-sectional imaging such as axial computed tomography and magnetic resonance, as well as plain radiographs.

Interpreting the image requires you to recognize the key organs or structures and orientate yourself with regards to the plane of imaging. Once you have worked out the plane of imaging, your brain will then help you identify anatomy you expect to be found based on your 3D anatomical map.

Reminder

Axial or transverse – cross-sectional images. Think of the old magician's trick of sawing someone in half. Imagine the patient's feet nearest to you, and the head furthest away with a pile of contiguous 'slices' available for you to scroll through. The right-sided structures are on the left-hand side of the image and vice versa.

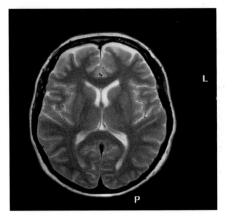

Axial Image, (L) = left, (P) = posterior

Coronal or frontal – the planes run from cephalad to caudad, separating the patient into front and back portions.

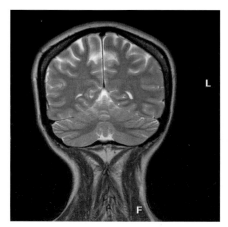

Coronal Image, (L) = left, (F) = frontal

Mid-sagittal – the plane divides the patient from cephalad to caudad but this time in an anterior to posterior direction through the midline.

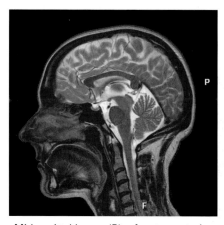

Mid-sagittal Image (P) refers to posterior

Purpose

This book displays radiological images with labels highlighting various organs and structures. Your aim is to identify the labelled anatomy and have a sound anatomical knowledge with respect to surgical practice. You are not expected to get all the answers correct first time around, so do not get despondent if you struggle.

Remember that the examiners use radiological imaging as a springboard to go on to discuss the relevant anatomy, which you should know. Mistakes with image interpretation are tolerated (you are not expected to be a radiologist) as long as the morbid and surgical anatomical knowledge is sound.

Vascular

Question 1.1

Name the structures labelled on this chest radiograph.

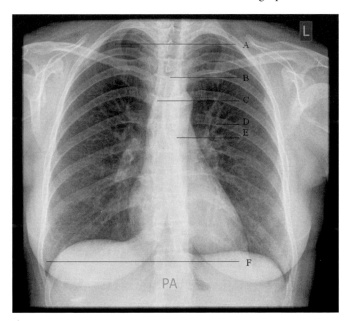

Figure 1.1

Answer
A: Right 1st rib.
B: Trachea.
C: Right main bronchus.
D: Posterior rib.
E: Left main bronchus.
F: Right costophrenic angle.

Anatomical notes

The thorax is divided into two lateral compartments each containing a lung and associated pleura, and a central compartment, the mediastinum, which contains the other thoracic structures. Each lung is surrounded by a pleural sac, created by two pleural membranes in close apposition. Pleural membranes:
- Visceral: lies in contact with the lung.
- Parietal: lies in contact with the diaphragm (innervated by vagus nerve), pericardium and chest wall (innervated by intercostals nerves).

The pleural cavities are potential spaces between the pleura and contain a layer of serous fluid that allows the layers to glide over each other during respiration. The parietal pleura produces pleural reflections as it changes direction. Reflections occur where the costal pleura becomes continuous with the mediastinal pleura anteriorly and posteriorly, and with the diaphragmatic pleura inferiorly. The visceral and parietal layers of pleura are continuous at the root of the lung. The pulmonary ligament, a double layer of parietal pleura, suspends from this region.

The lung root contains:
- Main bronchus.
- Pulmonary artery.
- Pulmonary vein.
- Bronchial arteries.
- Lymph nodes.

The **vagus nerve** runs **anterior** to the lung root, whereas the **phrenic nerve** runs **posterior** to this structure.

During expiration the lung does not completely occupy the thoracic cavity, creating potential pleural cavities.
- Costodiaphragmatic recess (diaphragmatic pleura in contact with costal pleura).
- Costomediastinal recess (posterior to the sternum).

Question 1.2

What type of image is shown below?
What thoracic level is it showing?
Name the labelled lobe/structure.

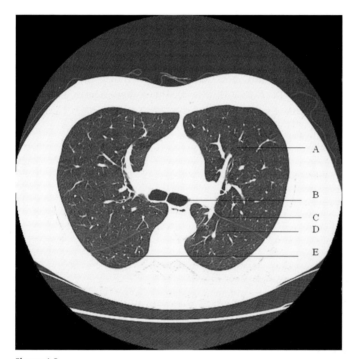

Figure 1.2

Answer
This is an axial lung CT (computed tomography) scan taken at the level of the
carina (T4/5).

A: Left upper lobe.
B: Left main bronchus.
C: Left oblique fissure.
D: Left lower lobe.
E: Right lower lobe.

Anatomical notes

The trachea begins at the level of C6 and continues inferiorly from the cricoid
cartilage to the carina (bifurcation) at the vertebral level of T4/5 (angle of

Louis). The right and left main bronchi pass inferolaterally from this level and branch within the lungs to form the bronchial tree, consisting of secondary (lobar) and tertiary (segmental) bronchi. Each bronchopulmonary segment has an apex that faces the root of the lung and a base at the pleural surface.

The right main bronchus is shorter, wider and leaves the main bronchus at a more vertical angle than the left main bronchus. The left main bronchus passes inferolaterally, inferior to the arch of aorta and anterior to the oesophagus and thoracic aorta to reach the root of the lung. C-shaped cartilage rings support the bronchi.

The right lung is divided into three lobes by the oblique and horizontal fissures. The left lung has two lobes, divided by the oblique fissure. Each lung has the following surfaces:
- Costal surface.
- Mediastinal.
- Diaphragmatic.

The lung borders are as follows:
- Anterior.
- Inferior.
- Posterior.

Clinical notes

Due to the vertical course and greater width of the right main bronchus there is a greater tendency for foreign bodies and aspirated material to pass into it.

Antoine Louis (1723–1792) – French surgeon and physiologist.

Question 1.3

Name the vascular structures identified on the chest radiograph.

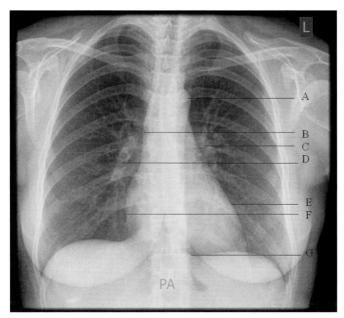

Figure 1.3

Answer
A: Aortic knuckle.
B: Superior vena cava (SVC).
C: Left pulmonary artery.
D: Right pulmonary artery.
E: Left heart border: left ventricle.
F: Right heart border: right atrium.
G: Inferior heart border: right ventricle.

Anatomical notes

The mediastinum is the central part of the thoracic cavity which lies between the pleural sacs. It extends from the superior thoracic aperture to the diaphragm and from the sternum and costal cartilages to the thoracic vertebrae. An arbitrary line formed between the sternal angle to the inferior border of T4 divides the mediastinum into superior and inferior parts. The inferior mediastinum is subdivided by the pericardium into anterior, middle and posterior parts. The heart and great vessels lie within the middle mediastinum.

The heart has a base, apex, three surfaces and four borders. The base of the heart is located posteriorly and formed mainly by the left atrium. The apex is normally located in the left fifth intercostal space, mid-clavicular line in adults and is formed by the left ventricle.

The three surfaces are:

- Sternocostal (right ventricle).
- Diaphragmatic (left ventricle and part of right ventricle).
- Pulmonary (left ventricle).

The borders comprise:

- Right heart border: formed by the right atrium and located between the superior and inferior vena cavae.
- Left heart border: formed by the left ventricle and partly by the left auricle.
- Superior border: formed by the right and left auricles.
- Inferior border: formed mainly by right ventricle, partly by left ventricle.

Question 1.4

What does the image below show?
Name the labelled structures.

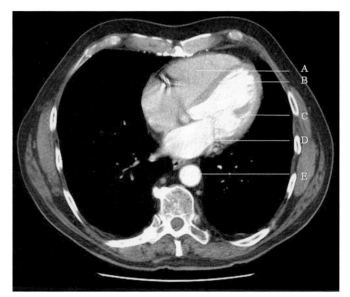

Figure 1.4

Answer
The image shows a CT axial slice through the thorax, demonstrating the
chambers of the heart.

A: Right ventricle.
B: Interventricular septum.
C: Left ventricle.
D: Left atrium.
E: Descending aorta.

Anatomical notes

The heart has four chambers: two atria and two ventricles. The right atrium
receives blood from the superior and inferior vena cavae, the coronary sinus
and anterior cardiac vein. The crista terminalis is a muscular ridge which runs
vertically downwards between the vena cavae and separates the smooth-walled
posterior part of the atrium (derived from the sinus venosus) from the

rough-walled anterior portion (derived from true fetal atrium). It is also the site of the sino-atrial node (SAN), the pacemaker of the heart.

The right ventricle is separated from the right atrium by the tricuspid valve and from the pulmonary trunk by the pulmonary valve. The inflow and outflow tracts of the ventricle are separated by a muscular ridge, the infundibuloventricular crest. The inner aspect of the inflow tract has a number of irregular muscular elevations (trabeculae carneae), whereas the outflow is smooth-walled. A muscular bundle, termed the moderator band, crosses the ventricular cavity from the interventricular septum to the anterior wall and conveys the right branch of the atrioventricular bundle.

The left atrium has thicker walls, but is smaller than the right. The pulmonary vein openings lie on its posterior wall, whereas the depression corresponding to the fossa ovalis of the right ventricle lies on the septal surface. The atrium communicates with the left ventricle via the mitral valve. The left ventricular wall is marked by thick trabeculae carnae, with the exception of the fibrous vestibule which lies immediately below the aortic orifice.

Question 1.5

What does the image show and can you name the labelled structures?

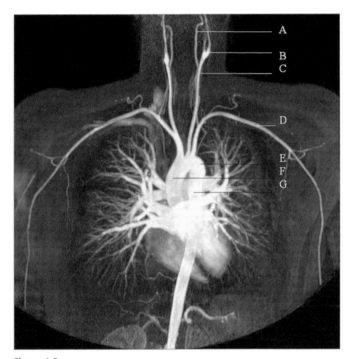

Figure 1.5

Answer

This is a coronal magnetic resonance angiographic image demonstrating the mediastinal aorta and its branches.

A: Left vertebral artery.
B: Common carotid artery bifurcation.
C: Left common carotid artery.
D: Left subclavian artery.
E: Arch of aorta.
F: Ascending aorta.
G: Descending aorta.

Anatomical notes

The arch of the aorta lies at approximately the level of T4. It gives rise to three main branches: the right brachiocephalic (inominate), the left common carotid and the left subclavian arteries. The right brachiocephalic artery divides into the right subclavian and the right common carotid arteries.

The common carotid artery ascends the neck in the carotid sheath lying medial to the internal jugular vein and anterior-medial to the vagus nerve. It terminates by division into the internal and external carotid arteries at approximately the level of C4. The internal carotid artery has no branches in the neck.

The vertebral arteries originate from the subclavian arteries. They ascend in the neck through the upper six foramina transversaria of the cervical spine. They converge at the junction between the medulla oblongata and the pons to form the basilar artery. (Refer to the neurosurgery chapter for a more detailed description of the cerebral circulation.)

Clinical notes

Occlusion of the subclavian artery proximal to the origin of the vertebral artery may result in compensatory retrograde blood flow in that vertebral artery. This has been termed the subclavian steal phenomenon.

Exercising the arm on the affected side results in a need for increased blood delivery. Since the subclavian artery is occluded the exercising arm achieves this requirement by 'stealing' the blood from the ipsilateral vertebral artery. This leaves the brain momentarily deficient of blood leading to transient neurological symptoms such as dizziness, unsteadiness, vertigo and visual disturbances. The combination of retrograde vertebral artery blood flow and neurological symptoms is termed **subclavian steal syndrome**.

Question 1.6

What does this image show and can you name the labelled structures?

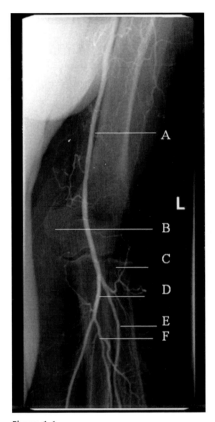

Figure 1.6

Answer
This is an angiogram of the left arm, demonstrating the brachial artery and its branches.

A: Brachial artery.
B: Medial epicondyle.
C: Radial head.
D: Ulnar artery.
E: Radial artery.
F: Anterior interosseous artery.

Anatomical notes

The brachial artery provides the arterial supply to the arm. It is a continuation of the axillary artery and begins at the lower border of teres major, and terminates by dividing into the ulnar and radial arteries at the level of the neck of the radius in the cubital fossa, under the cover of the bicipital aponeurosis.

It is a superficial structure that can be palpated throughout its course, lying anterior to triceps and brachialis, initially medial and then anterior to the humerus. As it passes inferolaterally the artery accompanies the median nerve, which crosses it from lateral to medial at the midpoint of the humerus.

In addition to the nutrient artery to the humerus, the brachial artery gives off three collateral branches:

- Profunda brachii.
- Superior and inferior ulnar collateral arteries.

The profunda brachii is given off high up in the arm to the extensor compartment where it runs with the radial nerve in the spiral groove of the humerus, before dividing into two terminal branches. These terminal branches, together with the ulnar collaterals, form an important anastomosis around the elbow joint with recurrent branches of the radial and ulnar arteries. The brachial artery is accompanied by paired venae commitantes.

Question 1.7

What radiological technique is being used here?
Name the labelled structures and the boundaries of the cubital fossa.

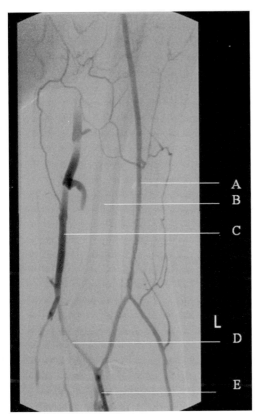

Figure 1.7

Answer
This is a venogram of the left arm.

A: Cephalic vein.
B: Humeral shaft.
C: Basilic vein.
D: Median cubital vein.
E: Median vein of forearm.

Anatomical notes

The cubital fossa is the hollow triangular space on the anterior surface of the elbow. Its boundaries are:

- Superiorly: an imaginary line connecting the medial and lateral epicondyles.
- Medially: pronator teres.
- Laterally: brachioradialis.
- Floor: brachialis and supinator.
- Roof: deep fascia that blends with the bicipital aponeurosis, superficial fascia and skin.

The contents of the cubital fossa are: the brachial artery and terminal branches, median cubital vein, median, radial and lateral antebrachial cutaneous nerves.

In the forearm the superficial veins (cephalic, median, basilic, and their connecting veins) make a variable, M-shaped pattern. The cephalic and basilic veins occupy the bicipital grooves, one on each side of biceps brachii.

Clinical notes

The cubital fossa is an important anatomical landmark for venepuncture. The bicipital aponeurosis separates the brachial artery from the median cubital vein. This was thought to be important when a patient underwent phlebotomy from the median cubital vein in former days as the bicipital aponeurosis protected the artery from the surgeon's knife and therefore gained the term: 'grâce à Dieu' (praise be to God).

Anatomy of the venous drainage of the arm and forearm is important, especially in fistula formation for haemodialysis: radio-cephalic, brachio-cephalic or basilic vein transposition.

Question 1.8

What anatomy does this angiogram demonstrate?
Name the labelled structures.

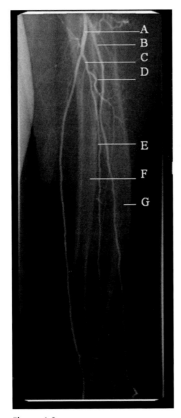

Figure 1.8

Answer
The angiogram demonstrates the branches of the radial and ulnar arteries

A: Ulnar artery.
B: Radial artery.
C: Common interosseous artery.
D: Posterior interosseous artery.
E: Anterior interosseous artery.
F: Ulnar.
G: Radius.

Anatomical notes

The ulnar and radial branches are terminal branches of the brachial artery and are formed opposite the neck of radius in the inferior part of the cubital fossa. The larger of the two branches is the ulnar artery which leaves the fossa deep to pronator teres and flexor digitorum superficialis, just lateral to the median nerve. It lies on flexor digitorum profundis and lateral to flexor carpi ulnaris before passing superficially to the flexor retinaculum.

At the level of pronator teres the ulnar artery gives off the common interosseous artery which divides into anterior and posterior interosseous arteries.

The radial artery arises in the cubital fossa and descends inferolaterally deep to brachioradialis, crossing anterior to the biceps tendon to lie on supinator. It then passes down the radial side of the forearm; lying on pronator teres, flexor digitorum superficialis, flexor pollicis longus and pronator quadrates before passing onto the lower end of the radius where its pulse is palpable lateral to the tendon of flexor carpi radialis.

Question 1.9

Name the vascular and bony labelled structures.
What is the clinical significance of the palmar arches?
What clinical test is performed to determine patency of the ulnar artery and how is it performed?

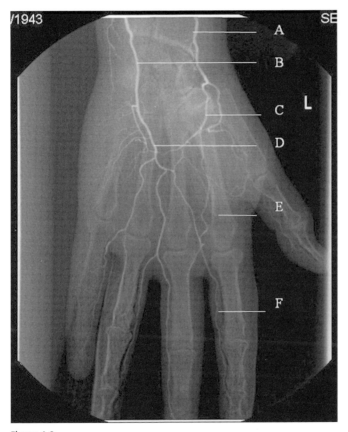

Figure 1.9

Answer
A: Radial artery.
B: Ulnar artery.
C: Deep palmar arch.
D: Superficial palmar arch.
E: Index metacarpal.
F: Digital artery.

Anatomical notes

The ulnar artery gives rise to the superficial palmar arch (most distal) which lies deep to the palmar aponeurosis. The deep palmar arch is derived from the radial artery after it pierces the first interosseous muscle. The superficial and deep arches are completed by communicating branches from the radial and ulnar arteries, respectively.

The superficial arch gives rise to palmar digital arteries to the little, ring and middle fingers, and the ulnar half of the index finger, whereas the deep arch gives rise to the palmar digital branches to the thumb and remaining half of the index finger (princeps pollicis and radialis indicis arteries). The dorsal arch also gives rise to three palmar metacarpal arteries which, after supplying the small muscles of the hand and the metacarpal bones, anastomose with the dorsal metacarpal arteries (these give rise to the dorsal digital arteries) which arise from the dorsal carpal arch.

Clinical notes

Allen's test is performed to test the patency of the radial and ulnar arteries. This is achieved by occluding the radial and ulnar arteries at the wrist, by direct pressure. The patient is then asked to open their hand which should be white. The pressure over the ulnar artery is released, whilst continuing to occlude the radial artery and the palm should become pink. The test is repeated again; this time releasing the radial artery and occluding the ulnar. If the palm does not become pink this signifies an occlusion of the released artery.

This is clinically important when planning surgical arteriovenous fistulae and radial artery donation for coronary artery bypass grafting.

Question 1.10

Name the labelled structures A–E.
At what vertebral level does letter B lie at?
Name the unpaired branches of the abdominal aorta and the vertebral levels
they leave the aorta.

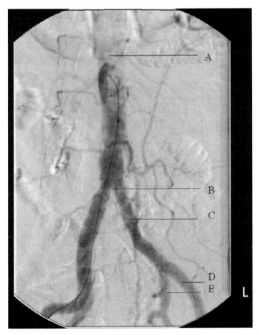

Figure 1.10a

Answer
A: Abdominal aorta.
B: Bifurcation of abdominal aorta (L4).
C: Left common iliac artery.
D: Left external iliac artery.
E: Left internal iliac artery.

Anatomical notes

The abdominal aorta is a continuation of the descending thoracic aorta, as it
passes through the diaphragm at the level of T12. It ends at L4 where it
bifurcates into the common iliac arteries. The branches of the abdominal
aorta are described as visceral or parietal and paired or unpaired:

Unpaired branches:
- Coeliac trunk (T12).
- Superior mesenteric artery (L1).
- Inferior mesenteric artery (L3).
  Paired visceral:
- Suprarenal.
- Renal.
- Gonadal.
  Paired parietal:
- Subcostal.
- Inferior phrenic.
- Lumbar.
  Unpaired parietal:
- Median sacral.

Clinical notes

Seventy-five per cent of abdominal aortic aneurysms are asymptomatic and often an incidental finding. The common presenting symptom is pain radiating into the back and flanks. Their complications are:

- Rupture: Intraperitoneal rupture causing exsanguination and shock, whereas a retroperitoneal bleed can be tamponaded by the surrounding tissues.
- Fistulation: Into bowel, IVC or left renal vein.
- Thrombosis: Leads to lower limb ischaemia.
- Distal embolism: May give rise to the clinical spectrum of acute ischaemia to trash foot.
- Distal obliteration: Patients may present with symptoms of distal occlusive disease such as claudication, rest pain or gangrene.

The risk of rupture increases with the size of the aneurysm. Surgeons or interventional radiologists would offer an elective repair or stent-grafting for aneurysms > 5.5 cm in diameter.

See figure opposite: this is a T2-weighted sagittal MR which shows an aortic aneurysm (white arrow).

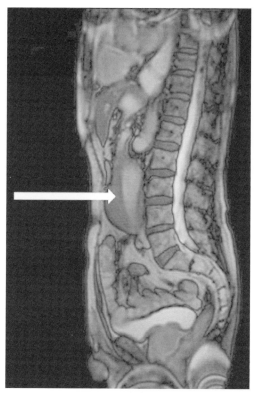

Figure 1.10b

Question 1.11

Name the arteries labelled on this angiogram.

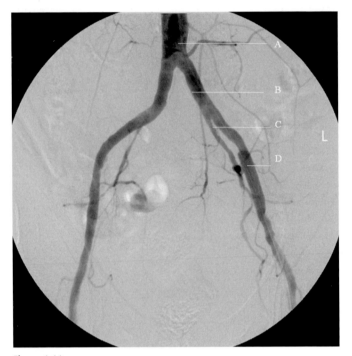

Figure 1.11

Answer

This is an iliac angiogram.

A: Abdominal aorta.
B: Left common iliac artery.
C: Left internal iliac artery.
D: Left external iliac artery.

Anatomical notes

The common iliac arteries commence at the bifurcation of the aorta, just to the left of the midline at L4. They pass inferolaterally and bifurcate anterior to the sacroiliac joint to give the external and internal iliac arteries.

The external iliac artery descends laterally from the common iliac artery to pass under the inguinal ligament at the mid-inguinal point where it becomes the femoral artery. The medial border of psoas major lies posterolaterally, whilst the femoral vein lies medially. Anteromedially, it is covered by peritoneum on which lies small bowel and sigmoid colon. It is crossed at its origin by the ureter and then by gonadal vessels, genital branch of the genitiofemoral nerve, deep circumflex iliac vein and vas deferens or round ligament.

Question 1.12

Name the labelled branches on this coeliac angiogram.
At which vertebral level does the coeliac axis leave the abdominal aorta?

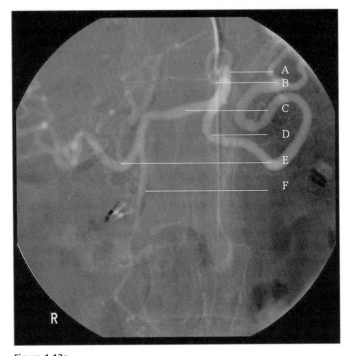

Figure 1.12a

Answer
A: Coeliac trunk.
B: Left gastric artery.
C: Common hepatic artery.
D: Splenic artery.
E: Common hepatic artery.
F: Gastroduodenal artery.

The coeliac axis leaves the aorta at the vertebral level of T12.

Anatomical notes

The coeliac axis supplies the embryological foregut and arises from the anterior aspect of the abdominal aorta at the level of the lower border of T12 and after 1 cm divides into its terminal branches:
- Left gastric artery.
- Splenic artery.
- Common hepatic artery.

Left gastric artery

This passes superolaterally on the posterior wall of the lesser sac to reach the gastro-oesophageal junction, where it divides into oesophageal branches. The terminal gastric branches anastomose with the right gastric artery.

Splenic artery

This passes laterally, to the left, and runs in the posterior wall of the lesser sac. It has a tortuous course which takes it along the superior border of the pancreas, anterior to left crus of diaphragm, upper pole of left kidney and adrenal gland before entering the lienorenal ligament to reach the splenic hilum.

Common hepatic artery

It passes inferolaterally to the right in the posterior wall of the lesser sac. It runs towards the first part of the duodenum and gives off the gastroduodenal and right gastric arteries. It then moves anteriorly as the hepatic artery to pass into the inferior margin of the opening of the lesser sac. It lies anterior to the portal vein, with the bile duct on its right as it ascends to terminate at the porta hepatis as the right and left hepatic branches (see Figure 1.12b).

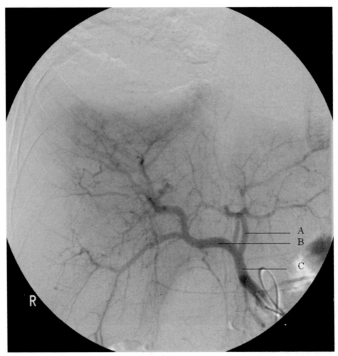

Figure 1.12b Hepatic angiogram. A, left hepatic artery; B, right hepatic artery; C, common hepatic artery.

Question 1.13

What radiological investigation does this image show?
Name the labelled anatomical structures.

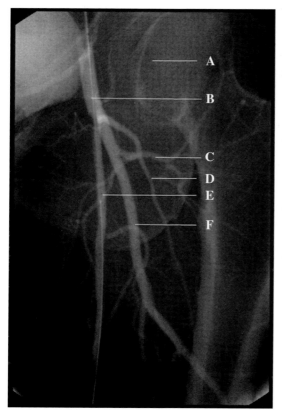

Figure 1.13

Answer
A lower limb angiogram has been performed, demonstrating branches of the left femoral artery.

A: Femoral head.
B: Common femoral artery.
C: Lateral circumflex femoral artery.
D: Descending branch.
E: Superficial femoral artery.
F: Profunda femoris.

Anatomical notes

The femoral artery is a direct continuation of the external iliac artery. It commences posterior to the inguinal ligament at the mid-inguinal point (half way between the anterior-superior iliac spine and the symphysis pubis) and ends as it passes through the adductor hiatus in adductor magnus to become the popliteal artery.

It has the following branches:

- Superficial epigastric.
- Superficial circumflex iliac.
- Superficial external pudendal.
- Deep external pudendal.
- Lateral circumflex femoral.
- Medial circumflex femoral.
- Profunda femoris.
- Descending genicular.
- Perforating branches.

Proximally it lies in the femoral sheath with the femoral vein medial to it. Lateral to it and outside the femoral sheath lies the femoral nerve. The artery lies on the tendon of psoas major and is separated from pectineus and adductor longus by the femoral vein which comes to lie progressively more posterior to the artery within the femoral triangle.

As the femoral artery enters the adductor canal it lies on adductor longus and then on adductor magnus, with vastus medialis lying anteriorly. Initially it is covered only by deep fascia then by sartorius.

The main branch of the femoral artery is the profunda femoris which is given off posterolaterally just below the femoral sheath, 3.5 cm below the inguinal ligament. It runs posteriorly between pectineus and adductor longus and passes deep into the thigh where it supplies the deep structures and posterior and medial compartments. The perforating and descending branches anastomose with the genicular branches of the popliteal artery.

Question 1.14

Label the anatomical structures demonstrated on this lower limb angiogram.
List the branches of structure C.

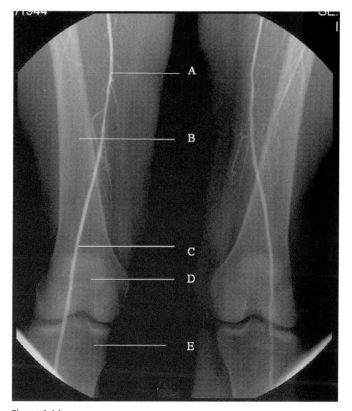

Figure 1.14

Answer
A: Superficial femoral artery.
B: Femoral shaft.
C: Popliteal artery.
D: Patella.
E: Medial tibial condyle.

Anatomical notes

The popliteal artery commences as the continuation of the femoral artery as it passes through the adductor hiatus and ends as it passes under the fibrous arch of soleus, immediately dividing into anterior and posterior tibial arteries. The popliteal artery extends from a hand's breadth above the knee and to the same distance below it.

On entering the popliteal fossa it lies medial to the femur and becomes the deepest structure, with only fat between it and the popliteal surface of the femur. More distally it lies on the capsule of the knee joint and then on popliteus. Initially biceps femoris is lateral to it and semimembranosus is medial. It then lies between the two heads of gastrocneumius. It is crossed laterally to medially by the tibial nerve and the popliteal vein with the vein always between the artery and nerve.

The branches of the popliteal artery are:
- Superior medial and lateral geniculate arteries.
- Middle genicular artery.
- Inferior medial and lateral geniculate arteries.
- Anterior and posterior tibial arteries.
- Muscular branches.

Clinical notes

The popliteal artery is a site of aneurysms. They are commonest in men and those over the age of 50. Atherosclerosis is the commonest cause, but others include: collagen disorders, fibromuscular dysplasia, infection, or blunt and penetrating trauma.

Complications of popliteal artery aneurysms are:
- Rupture.
- Acute occlusion and lower limb ischaemia.
- Tibial nerve compression.
- Popliteal vein thrombosis.

Question 1.15

Below is an angiogram demonstrating the leg vessels.
Name the structures labelled A-F.

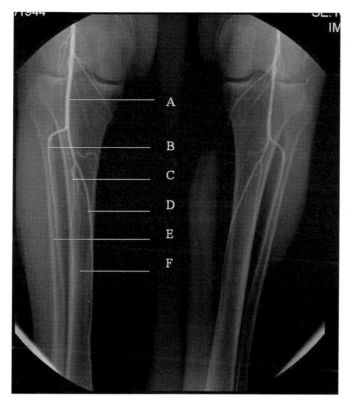

Figure 1.15

Answer
A: Popliteal artery.
B: Anterior tibial artery.
C: Peroneal artery.
D: Posterior tibial artery.
E: Shaft of fibula.
F: Shaft of tibia.

Anatomical notes

The anterior tibial artery commences at the bifurcation of the popliteal artery just under the fibrous arch of soleus and supplies the structures in the extensor compartment of the leg. It passes anteriorly between the heads of tibialis posterior and descends on the interosseous membrane to cross the lower tibia at the ankle joint, midway between the malleoli. Here it continues over the dorsum of the foot as the dorsalis pedis artery, gives off the arcuate artery, and runs between the 1st and 2nd metatarsals to join the lateral plantar artery in the formation of the plantar arch.

The posterior tibial artery is the largest terminal branch of the popliteal artery and supplies the structures of the posterior compartment of the leg. It descends deep to soleus, lying on tibialis posterior, flexor digitorum longus, the tibia and ankle joint. It passes behind the medial malleolus between the tendons of flexor digitorum longus and flexor hallucis longus, accompanied by the posterior tibial vein and tibial nerve. Below the ankle it divides into the medial and lateral plantar arteries, which supply the foot.

2

General surgery and urology

Question 2.1

Can you identify the labelled anatomy on this supine abdominal radiograph?

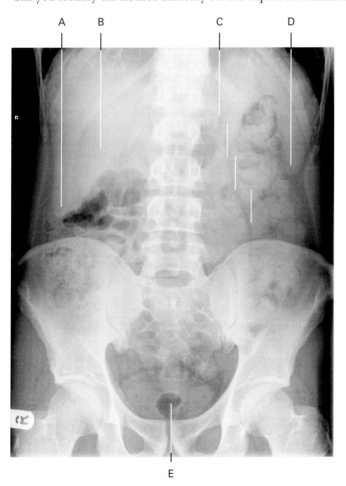

Figure 2.1

Answer
A: Tip of right lobe of liver.
B: Right kidney.
C: Left psoas shadow.
D: Tip of spleen.
E: Rectum.

Anatomical notes

The liver occupies the right hypochondrium. Traditionally it is divided into left and right lobes by the falciform ligament antero-superiorly and the fissures of ligamentum teres and ligamentum venosum posteriorly. The liver can be further subdivided into eight segments, each with a separate blood supply and biliary drainage. The left and right branches of the hepatic portal vein and the three hepatic veins form useful landmarks and boundaries for describing segmental liver anatomy on imaging.

The spleen typically occupies the left hypochondrium and measures up to 12 cm in cranio-caudal length. It is often not identified on a plain abdominal radiograph but surrounding fat, as in this example, may outline its inferior tip.

The lateral aspect of the left psoas muscle is also well demonstrated due to adjacent fat. The right psoas border is not as clear in this example, because of overlying bowel gas.

Clinical notes

Plain film radiography of the abdomen is particularly useful as initial imaging if bowel obstruction is being considered. Distended gas-filled bowel is usually well demonstrated. However, if the obstructed bowel is fluid filled it may not be clearly identified on plain film. Computed tomography is the investigation of choice if there is ongoing clinical concern.

The jejunum is typically found to the left of the midline and towards the hypochondrium; a transverse lumen diameter over 3.5 cm is considered abnormal. The ileum is typically found to the right of the midline and towards the iliac fossa; a diameter over 2.5 cm is abnormal. The jejunum typically has a higher concentration of valvulae conniventes than the ileum. This increase in mucosal surface area befits the jejunum's role as the predominant absorbing portion of the small bowel.

Gas-filled colon can usually be differentiated from small bowel on a plain radiograph by the presence of haustra. These projections into the lumen can be seen as linear areas perpendicular to the length of the colon wall, but only partially traverse the width of the lumen. Valvulae conniventes in small bowel on the other hand are seen to pass all the way across the lumen.

Question 2.2

This is a CT axial section of the upper abdomen. Can you name the labelled structures?

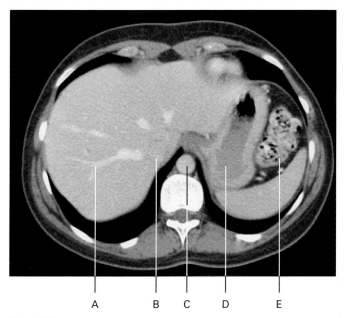

Figure 2.2

Answer
A: Right hepatic vein.
B: Inferior vena cava.
C: Descending aorta.
D: Stomach.
E: Splenic flexure of colon.

Anatomical notes

There are three hepatic veins (right, middle and left), which drain blood away from the liver, into the inferior vena cava (IVC).

The diaphragmatic foramen of the IVC is located at the level of the 8th thoracic vertebral body. The IVC is accompanied by terminal branches of the right phrenic nerve.

The oesophageal hiatus is located at the level of the 10th thoracic vertebral body. The oesophagus is accompanied by the vagus nerves, oesophageal lymphatics and oesophageal branches of the left gastric vessels.

The diaphragmatic foramen of the aorta is located at the level of the 12th thoracic vertebral level. The aorta is accompanied by the azygos vein and thoracic duct.

Clinical notes

A hiatus hernia is generally considered to be a protrusion of any portion of the stomach into the thoracic cavity through the oesophageal hiatus. Sliding hiatus hernias are by far the most common and the gastro-oesophageal junction is typically displaced at least a centimetre above the level of the diaphragmatic hiatus. The hiatus itself may be abnormally widened. There is a somewhat complex relationship with lower oesophageal sphincter incompetence and gastro-oesophageal reflux disease. Many patients with large hernias are asymptomatic. Those who are symptomatic, however, may benefit from a fundoplication procedure, which can usually be performed laparoscopically.

Para-oesophageal hiatus hernias occur when the gastro-oesophageal junction remains below the hiatus, but a portion of stomach rolls up alongside it into the thoracic cavity. Mixed hiatal hernias consist of a gastro-oesophageal junction within the thorax and an associated para-oesophageal hernia. Large para-oesophageal hernias with abnormally rotated stomach are at risk of volvulus with obstruction and ischaemia.

Question 2.3

Name the investigation and identify the labelled anatomical regions or structures.

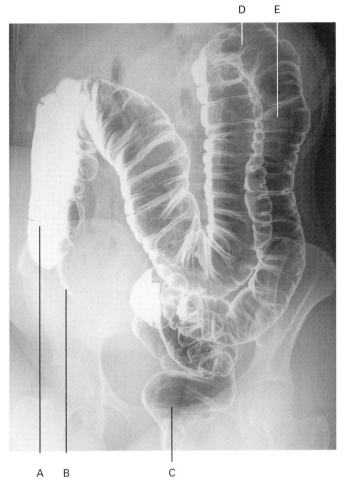

Figure 2.3

Answer
This is a double contrast barium enema.

A: Caecum.
B: Appendix.
C: Rectum.
D: Splenic flexure.
E: Descending colon.

Anatomical notes

Use the familiar bony anatomy to orientate yourself. The large intestine consists of the caecum, ascending colon, hepatic flexure, transverse colon, splenic flexure, descending colon, sigmoid colon, rectum and anal canal. Its length is highly variable but is said to average 1.5 metres in the adult.

The small bowel terminates at the ileocaecal valve, usually found at the medial aspect of the caecum. The lumen of the gastrointestinal tract can dramatically change at this point from a terminal ileal diameter of 2.5 cm to a caecal diameter of up to 9 cm. As well as a change in diameter there are three other morphological differences between small and large bowel:

1. **Appendices epiploicae**. Numerous fat-filled peritoneal structures known as appendices epiploicae are found covering the outer surface of the ascending, transverse and descending portions of the colon.
2. **Taeniae coli**. Three distinct bands formed from the condensed bulk of longitudinal muscle stretch from the base of the appendix along the length of the large bowel to the rectosigmoid junction.
3. **Sacculations**. These are baggy sac-like pouches and are formed because the taeniae coli are shorter than the natural length of the large bowel. Haustra are infoldings of the wall, which periodically project into the lumen. They are elegantly demonstrated by a barium enema study, and are not seen to completely span the diameter of the lumen in contradistinction to small bowel valvulae conniventes.

The appendix is again highly variable in length but consistently arises from the posteromedial aspect of the caecum typically just caudad to the ileocaecal valve. The lie of the appendix is also highly variable but the majority are situated retrocaecally.

The arterial blood supply of the large bowel arises from both the superior mesenteric artery (SMA) and inferior mesenteric artery (IMA). From the SMA the ileocolic artery supplies the caecum, the right colic artery supplies the ascending colon and the middle colic artery supplies the proximal two-thirds of the transverse colon. An appendicular branch of the ileocolic artery supplies the appendix. The IMA gives off a left colic branch to supply the distal one-third of transverse colon, the splenic flexure and descending colon. The IMA is also responsible for several sigmoid branches supplying the lower descending colon and sigmoid, and the superior rectal artery.

Clinical notes

Bowel preparation is essential to ensure a clean mucosa free from faecal matter, which would otherwise either obscure, or be confused with lesions on imaging. Barium is administered via a rectal catheter and coats the mucosa of the large bowel. Insufflating air and distending the large bowel lumen provides a double contrast effect. Bowel wall spasm prevents adequate visualization and a smooth muscle relaxant such as buscopan is administered, provided there are no contraindications. Polyps, tumours and other pathologies such as diverticular disease, which distort the mucosal lining, are well demonstrated.

Computed tomography colonography is being increasingly utilized as an alternative to barium enema examinations and conventional colonoscopy. Advantages include depiction of the whole bowel wall rather than just the lumen and the potential for identifying incidental or alternative extra-colonic pathology.

Colonoscopy has the advantage of allowing tissue biopsy for pathological examination, and is a radiation-free procedure. Although rare, the possibility of an iatrogenic bowel wall perforation is obviously the major potential disadvantage.

Understanding the arterial blood supply of the large bowel has particular clinical relevance when faced with a patient with possible bowel ischaemia. The SMA supplies the proximal two-thirds of the transverse colon via the middle colic artery. The IMA supplies the distal one-third of transverse colon (splenic flexure) and descending colon via the left colic artery. This arterial transition point just proximal to the splenic flexure is a watershed area, and is particularly prone to ischaemic damage.

Question 2.4

This is a T2-weighted magnetic resonance axial cross-section image of a male pelvis at the level of the rectum. Can you name the labelled structures?

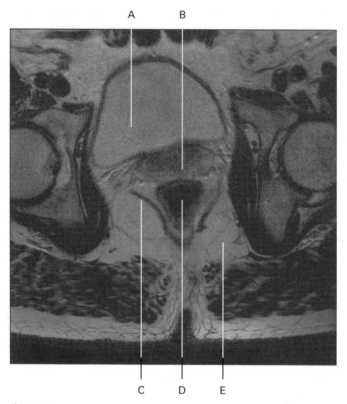

Figure 2.4

Answer
A: Bladder.
B: Prostate gland or peri-prostatic tissue.
C: Right levator ani muscle.
D: Lumen of rectum.
E: Left ischiorectal fossa.

Anatomical notes

The femoral heads, acetabulae and natal cleft should have helped you to orientate yourself. The adult rectum is approximately 12 cm long. The anal canal is inferior to the rectum and measures approximately 4 cm in length. The superior rectal artery is a branch of the IMA. The middle rectal artery arises from the internal iliac artery and the inferior rectal artery is a branch of the internal pudendal artery.

The dentate or pectinate line is a level that divides the superior and inferior anal canal. The superior rectal vein drains the rectum and anus above the dentate line into the portal venous circulation. The middle and inferior rectal veins drain the lower anal canal (below the dentate line) into the systemic circulation.

At the level of the dentate line the columnar epithelium lining the upper half of the anal canal changes to stratified squamous epithelium which lines the lower half. Lymphatic drainage above the line is to the internal iliac nodes whereas below the line the drainage is to the superficial inguinal nodes.

Clinical notes

The upper anal canal is innervated by the autonomic nervous system. Banding or injecting haemorrhoids above the dentate line is a pain-free procedure. Below the dentate line, however, the innervation is somatic, via the inferior rectal nerve, a branch of the pudendal nerve. If the doctor strays below the dentate line when banding or injecting sclerosant, the unwitting patient will be left in excruciating pain and the red-faced doctor will be left with some explaining to do.

The mucosal histology differences lend to a predilection of adenocarcinomas above the dentate line (columnar epithelium), and squamous cell carcinomas below the dentate line (stratified squamous epithelium).

Question 2.5

This is an axial CT section through the abdomen. Can you identify the labelled structures?

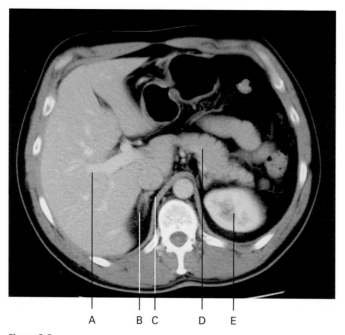

A   B C   D   E

Figure 2.5

Answer

A: Right portal vein.
B: Right adrenal gland (wishbone shaped).
C: Right crus of diaphragm.
D: Body of pancreas.
E: Upper pole of left kidney.

Anatomical notes

The portal venous system drains blood to the liver from the gastrointestinal tract, pancreas, gallbladder and spleen. The distal branches of the portal venous system mirror the terminal branches of the coeliac axis vessels, SMA and IMA. Proximally, however, the inferior mesenteric vein drains into the splenic vein behind the body of the pancreas. The proximal continuation of this vessel continues to be referred to as the splenic vein until the superior mesenteric vein enters it behind the head/neck of the pancreas. Beyond this confluence, the vessel is known as the portal vein. The portal vein courses deep to the duodenum and enters the liver at the porta hepatis.

The portal vein divides into right and left main branches within the liver and these branches further subdivide until eventually, terminal portal venules are formed. These drain into the sinusoids where portal venous blood is mixed with hepatic arterial inflow. Hepatic venous blood is then drained via branches which eventually form the three main hepatic veins, themselves draining into the IVC.

Clinical notes

Obstruction of the drainage of portal venous blood may occur for a number of congenital or acquired reasons. A consequent rise in portal venous blood pressure is known as portal hypertension. A simple and logical way of addressing the causes for portal hypertension (at least for viva purposes) is to group them into pre-hepatic, hepatic and post-hepatic.

Pre-hepatic causes include portal vein thrombosis, extrinsic compression from tumour or congenital obliteration. Hepatic causes include vascular fibrosis associated with cirrhosis and parasitic infection such as schistosomiasis. Post-hepatic causes include hepatic venous thrombosis and congenital webs causing hepatic vein or IVC obstruction. Post-hepatic venous outflow obstruction due to any cause that results in a secondary hepatic arterial or portal venous inflow problem is known as Budd–Chiari syndrome.

Portal hypertension results in the opening up of collateral pathways between the portal venous system and systemic circulation. The most clinically important collaterals to be aware of are oesophageal varices, which may cause acute and massive haematemesis. The communications exist between the oesophageal branches of the left gastric veins (portal venous) and the oesophageal veins of the azygos system (systemic venous).

Question 2.6

Can you identify the labelled anatomical structures?

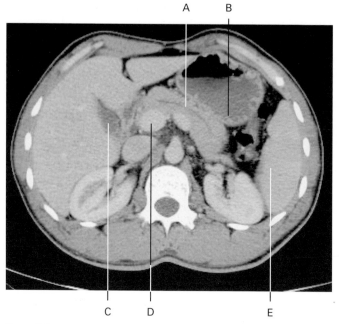

Figure 2.6

Answer
A: Pancreatic duct.
B: Gastric wall or rugal fold.
C: Gallbladder.
D: Splenoportal confluence.
E: Spleen.

Anatomical notes

The pancreas is retroperitoneal and ascends obliquely from the organ's head at the level of the first lumbar vertebral body to the tail at the level of the 12th thoracic vertebral body. The gland passes across the transpyloric plane of Addison. The head sits in the concavity created by the curve of the duodenum and the tail often reaches the splenic hilum. For descriptive purposes the pancreas also has a neck and body. The uncinate process projects from the head and curves posteriorly behind the superior mesenteric vessels.

The great vessels (IVC and aorta) lie deep to the head and neck of the pancreas. The portal vein commences once the superior mesenteric vein joins with the splenic vein at the portosplenic confluence. The coeliac axis and SMA arise from the aorta deep to the neck of the pancreas. The crura of the diaphragm lie anterolaterally in relation to the vertebral body. The left kidney lies deep to the pancreatic tail. The splenic vein also receives the inferior mesenteric vein just behind the tail, prior to it coursing to the confluence.

The common bile duct passes either just behind, or through the head of pancreas to join the pancreatic duct at the ampulla of Vater in the second part of the duodenum. As can be seen in the figure, the stomach is the major anterior relation of the pancreas although the two are separated to a variable extent by the lesser sac.

Arterial blood supply to the pancreas comes from the splenic artery and pancreaticoduodenal artery. The corresponding veins drain into the portal venous system.

Clinical notes

A neoplasm within the pancreatic head can cause obstructive jaundice due to mass effect with compression of the common bile duct. Most pancreatic tumours relate to the exocrine portion of the gland and are ductal adenocarcinomas. Endocrine neoplasms or islet cell tumours may be functioning, and release hormones such as gastrin or insulin. Non-functioning islet cell tumours do not release hormones.

Functioning islet cell tumours often present relatively early, due to the symptoms associated with the systemic effects of raised hormone levels. Examples include a gastrin-secreting gastrinoma, predisposing to refractory gastric ulcer disease, and an insulin-secreting insulinoma causing recurrent hypoglycaemic episodes.

The transpyloric plane of Addison is a horizontal (axial) line across the abdomen generally taken to be halfway between the suprasternal notch and the pubic symphysis. Organs and structures typically found along this plane include:
- The pylorus of the stomach.
- L1 vertebral body.
- Neck of pancreas.
- Portosplenic confluence.
- Renal hila.
- Fundus of gallbladder.
- Origin of SMA.
- Duodeno-jejunal flexure.

Lord Christopher Addison (1869–1951) Professor of Anatomy, University College, Sheffield. Also the first Minister of Health, 1919.

Question 2.7

What investigation has been performed? Can you identify the labelled anatomy?

A   B

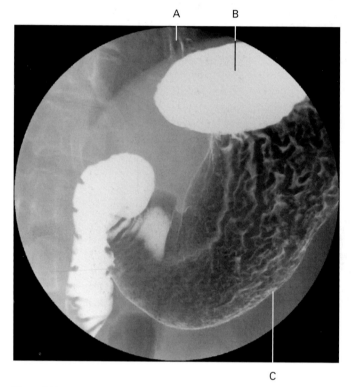

C

Figure 2.7

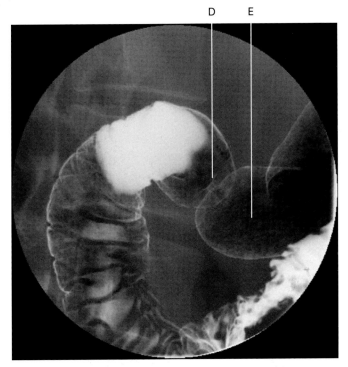

Figure 2.7

Answer

This is a barium meal.

A: Lower oesophagus.
B: Gastric fundus.
C: Greater curve of stomach.
D: Pylorus.
E: Gastric antrum.

Anatomical notes

The size of the stomach varies between individuals. It is a distensible muscular sac and its volume is dependent at any given time on gastric contents. Food is received from the oesophagus through the cardiac orifice at the gastro-oesophageal junction (GOJ). The stomach lies to the left of the midline and is J-shaped, with a lesser curve medially and a greater curve laterally. The fundus of the stomach is found above the level of the cardia, the region just distal to the

GOJ, and in close proximity to the heart. Distal to the cardia the major portion of stomach is known as the body, this in turn ends at the antrum, which is also known as the prepyloric region. The pylorus is a focal area of thickened circular gastric wall muscle, which acts as a sphincter to control gastric outlet.

Both the anterior and posterior walls of the stomach are covered in peritoneum. The peritoneum is continued from the lesser curve border to the liver as the lesser omentum. The peritoneum from the greater curve is continued as the greater omentum. The stomach is an anterior structure, and although the lesser curve may be covered by the left lobe of liver and the fundus by the diaphragm, the majority of the anterior surface lies just deep to the abdominal wall. The posterior relations of the stomach include the lesser sac, pancreas and spleen.

The arterial supply to the stomach is abundant with extensive arcades. Supply is from the left and right gastric arteries, the left and right gastro-epiploic arteries and the short gastric arteries.

- Left gastric artery arises directly from the coeliac axis.
- Right gastric artery arises from the hepatic artery.
- Left gastro-epiploic artery arises from the splenic artery.
- Right gastro-epiploic artery arises from the gastroduodenal artery.
- Short gastric arteries also arise from the splenic artery.

Clinical notes

An eroding posterior gastric ulcer in the body of the stomach can ulcerate into the splenic artery causing catastrophic haemorrhage. Similarly a posterior eroding ulcer in the prepyloric region can ulcerate into the gastroduodenal artery.

Barium swallow examinations are on the decline; the technique is being increasingly supplanted by upper gastrointestinal flexible endoscopy. Endoscopy also allows close examination of the mucosal surface but has the advantage of facilitating tissue biopsy for diagnostic purposes. Endoscopic ultrasound has a role in evaluating early gastric tumours but CT is established as the investigation of choice for staging gastric malignancy.

Question 2.8

Can you name the labelled anatomical structures or spaces?

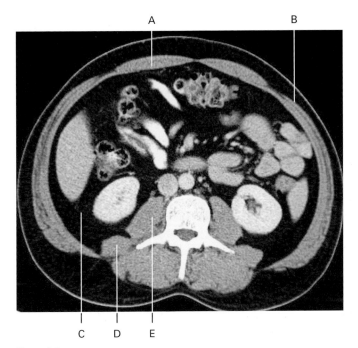

Figure 2.8

Answer
A: Rectus abdominis.
B: Left external oblique.
C: Pouch of Morison.
D: Right quadratus lumborum.
E: Right psoas major.

Regarding axial imaging of the abdomen: if no ribs are present and the iliac crest has not yet come into view, there is a good chance that you are at the level of the third lumbar vertebral body (L3).

Anatomical notes

The anterior abdominal wall musculature can be found deep to the skin, subcutaneous fat and Scarpa's fascia. The rectus abdominis muscles are a constant finding along the central anterior abdominal wall. They originate from the medial aspects of the 5th, 6th and 7th costal cartilages bilaterally and run longitudinally within the rectus sheath, to insert onto the pubic crest. The rectus sheath itself is formed from the aponeuroses of external oblique, internal oblique and transverses abdominis. The linea alba is the fusion of the aponeuroses in the midline.

Above the costal margin the external oblique muscle is the sole contributor of an aponeurotic layer to the rectus sheath. The external oblique muscles originate from the outer surfaces of the lower eight ribs and the iliac crest. The free lower border of external oblique forms the inguinal ligament, between the anterior superior iliac spine and pubic tubercle.

Below the costal margin, but above the level of the umbilicus (Figure 2.8) the external oblique and anterior leaf of the internal oblique aponeuroses form the anterior rectus sheath. The posterior rectus sheath is formed from the posterior leaf of the internal oblique and the transversus abdominis aponeuroses.

Below a point halfway between the umbilicus and pubis (arcuate line) all the aponeuroses pass in front of the rectus muscles to form a condensed fusion of all aponeuroses anteriorly. The posterior rectus sheath at this level is formed by default by the transversalis fascia and peritoneum.

Three transverse tendinous intersections fuse the anterior rectus sheath to the rectus muscles at specific locations: the xiphoid, umbilicus and halfway between these points.

Clinical notes

The inguinal canal allows the passage of the spermatic cord or round ligament through the lower abdominal wall. The canal passes obliquely, inferiorly and medially from the deep ring to the superficial ring. The deep ring is an opening in the transversalis fascia located halfway between the anterior superior iliac spine and pubic tubercle. The inferior epigastric vessels pass just medial to it. The superficial ring is a defect in the external oblique aponeurosis, above the pubic tubercle.

The anterior wall of the inguinal canal is predominantly formed from the external oblique muscle. The internal oblique also contributes to the lateral third of the anterior wall of the canal. The internal oblique and transversus abdominis muscles form the roof of the canal. The transversalis fascia forms the lateral portion of the posterior wall, with the conjoint tendon making up the medial aspect. The conjoint tendon is the combined common insertion of the transversus abdominis and internal oblique muscles. The floor of the inguinal canal is formed from the inguinal ligament (the free lower border of external oblique).

Indirect inguinal hernias pass through the deep inguinal ring and along the inguinal canal to emerge through the superficial ring and down into the scrotum in the male. Direct inguinal hernias, on the other hand, originate through a weakness in the posterior wall of the inguinal canal, rather than the deep ring. They too pass down the canal but rarely pass through the superficial ring. Once an inguinal hernia is reduced the examining clinician can test to see if it is direct or indirect. Compression over the deep ring will prevent increased abdominal pressure from causing an indirect hernia to protrude. The origin of a direct hernia will however be located medially to the deep ring and protrusion despite compression will occur. How does the clinician find the deep ring? This bit is easy. It is about a centimetre above the point where the femoral artery passes under the inguinal ligament. Palpate the femoral artery in the groin crease, and you have found your landmark. Press just above the inguinal ligament once the hernia is reduced. Do not forget that you have the anterior superior iliac spine and pubic tubercle to tell you where to find the ligament. The neck of a direct inguinal hernia is often wide and these hernias rarely strangulate.

James Rutherford Morison (1853–1939) British surgeon who named the hepatorenal pouch.

Question 2.9

What investigation has been performed? Can you identify the labelled structures?

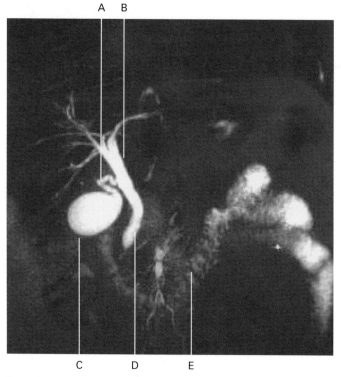

Figure 2.9

Answer

This is a magnetic resonance cholangiopancreatogram (MRCP).

A: Cystic duct.
B: Common hepatic duct.
C: Gallbladder.
D: Common bile duct.
E: Duodenum.

Anatomical notes

The biliary tree drains bile from hepatocytes into the gallbladder. Hormonal stimulation in the form of cholecystokinin (CCK) causes the gallbladder wall smooth muscle to contract and bile is then expelled into the duodenum to assist with the emulsification of fat.

Within the liver, the left and right main hepatic ducts join to form the common hepatic duct (CHD). The CHD descends inferiorly from the porta hepatis and is joined by the cystic duct to form the common bile duct (CBD). The cystic duct drains the gallbladder. The common bile duct then descends either just posterior to, or sometimes through, the pancreatic head to drain into the duodenum at the ampulla of Vater. The pancreatic duct usually joins the CBD at this point in the second part of the duodenum.

Clinical notes

The chief component of most gallstones is cholesterol. Supersaturation of bile with cholesterol leads to cholesterol crystal formation and aggregation, a precursor step to gallstone formation. Gallstones are present asymptomatically in many individuals, however they may act as the underlying aetiology for a whole range of conditions, which you should be able to comfortably discuss in a viva. Biliary colic, cholecystitis, pancreatitis, ascending cholangitis and gallstone ileus are the main pathologies in order of ascending morbidity.

The management of a patient with gallstones should include the offer of a laparoscopic cholecystectomy, whereby the gallbladder is dissected from its bed and the cystic artery and cystic duct are identified and clipped before dissection and removal. Many authorities advocate on-table cholangiograms (OTC) to confirm that there are no remnant intraductal calculi. Retained CBD stones post cholecystectomy are a cause of recurrent pain and jaundice, with the risks of ascending cholangitis and pancreatitis. Post cholecystectomy pain, especially with an obstructive picture on liver function biochemistry, is one of the indications for MRCP.

Question 2.10

This is a magnetic resonance angiogram of the kidneys. Can you identify the labelled anatomy?

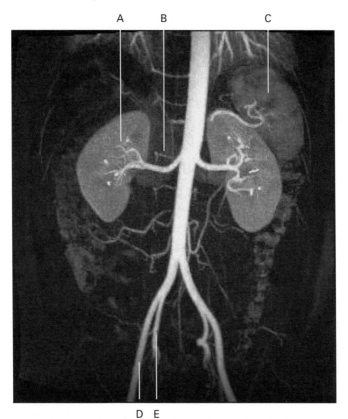

Figure 2.10a

Answer

A: Interlobar artery.
B: One of numerous lumbar arteries.
C: Spleen.
D: External iliac artery.
E: Internal iliac artery.

Anatomical notes

The kidneys are retroperitoneal organs situated posteriorly and laterally within the abdomen with their hila facing the midline great vessels. They lie against the posterior abdominal wall in an oblique position parallel to psoas major. They are generally located between the 12th thoracic vertebral body and the 3rd lumbar vertebral body level. The right kidney is slightly caudad when compared with the left due to the presence of the liver superiorly. At each hilum the renal artery enters and the renal vein and ureter exit the kidney. The ureter commences at the renal pelvis, and is the most posterior of the hila structures.

The posterior relations of the kidney are principally the diaphragm and costodiaphragmatic recesses of the pleura superiorly, quadratus lumborum laterally and psoas major medially. Superiorly the kidneys are in close relation to the adrenal (suprarenal) glands. The anterior surface of the left kidney is in close contact with the splenorenal ligament which contains the tail of pancreas and splenic vessels. The stomach and splenic flexure of colon as well as jejunum are also anterior relations of the left kidney. The liver is a major anterior relation of the right kidney, although the two are separated by the peritoneum of the hepatorenal pouch of Morison. The ascending colon and second part of duodenum are also major anterior relations of the right kidney.

Conventional renal angiogram

The renal arteries usually arise from the abdominal aorta somewhere between the L1 and L2 level. The aorta lies to the left of the midline necessitating a right renal artery which is longer than its left-sided counterpart. The right renal artery passes behind the IVC on its way to the hilum.

The main renal artery usually divides as soon as it enters the hilum with branches to the upper and lower portions of the organ. The kidney has five segments each with their own arterial supply, but no collateral circulation. Interlobar arteries pass between the renal pyramids through the renal columns. Arcuate arteries are given off at the corticomedullary junction and these traverse along this plane giving off interlobular arteries into the renal cortex which eventually divide down to afferent arterioles. Distal to the glomeruli, efferent arterioles form a secondary arterial bed to supply the convoluted tubules downstream. The draining veins parallel the course of the arteries and eventually anastomose to form the main renal vein.

The kidney benefits from a smooth, true fibrous capsule superficial to the cortex, which surrounds and protects it. The kidneys are also surrounded by

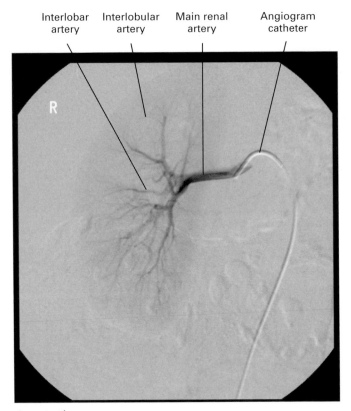

Figure 2.10b

perirenal fat which separates them from other abdominal organs and the suprarenal glands. This perirenal fat is in turn surrounded by a condensation of fascia. This fascia conveniently divides the retroperitoneum into three separate spaces. The perirenal space is the space immediately surrounding the kidney and is bound by the renal fascia. The anterior and posterior pararenal spaces lie anterior and posterior to the renal fascia. The renal fascia itself is formed from an anterior layer known as the Gerota's fascia and a posterior layer known as Zuckerkandl's fascia. These layers are fused where they join laterally and are then referred to as the lateral conal fasciae. They become continuous with the deep fascia of the abdomen.

Clinical notes

Magnetic resonance angiography of the kidneys is often requested to assess a patient with refractory hypertension who is suspected of having renovascular disease. The main cause in the young is fibromuscular dysplasia, whereas in the elderly population atherosclerosis is the chief culprit. Both conditions cause renal hypoperfusion and subsequent activation of the rennin-angiotensin-aldosterone mechanism to facilitate an unnecessary increase in systolic blood pressure. Treatment is predominantly endovascular with angioplasty, and if necessary stenting.

Dimitrie Gerota (1867–1939) Romanian anatomist.

Emil Zuckerkandl (1849–1910) Austro-Hungarian anatomist.

Question 2.11

This is a T2-weighted mid-sagittal image of the female pelvis. Can you name the labelled anatomy? What is the normal variant?

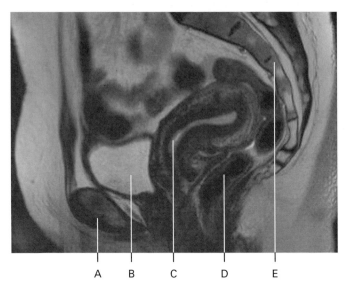

A   B   C   D   E

Figure 2.11

Answer
A: Pubic symphysis.
B: Bladder.
C: Endometrium of uterus.
D: Rectum.
E: Coccyx.

Normal variant = retroverted uterus.

Anatomical and clinical notes

Knowledge of rectal anatomy is a vital prerequisite to understanding the principles of surgery for rectal cancer. En-bloc removal of the rectum and adjacent lymph nodes in a total mesorectal excision has been shown to reduce the risk of disease recurrence. The rectum is surrounded by its own mesorectal fascia. Posterior to this lies a potential retrorectal space, which is limited posteriorly by the presacral parietal fascia. The presacral fascia overlies the presacral vessels anterior to the sacrum and coccyx. Posterior extension of a rectal tumour may cause sciatica by involving the lower sacral nerves, which emerge from the anterior sacral foramina.

Anteriorly, the upper two-thirds of the rectum are covered by peritoneum, which extends posteriorly from the uppermost posterior surface of the bladder. A recess between the bladder and rectum, lined by peritoneum is known as the rectovesical pouch in males. A rectouterine pouch of Douglas is the equivalent in females. Anterior relations of the lower third of rectum in the male include the prostate, base of bladder and seminal vesicles. The vagina is the main anterior relation of the lower third of rectum in the female. The rectum is separated from anterior structures by a layer of fascia known as Denonvilliers, which forms the anterior surface of the mesorectum. Laterally the rectum is supported by the levator ani muscles. The operating surgeon must identify the correct fascial planes prior to attempting a full dissection.

Dr James Douglas (1675–1742) Scottish anatomist.

Charles Pierre Denonvilliers (1808–1872) Professor of Anatomy and Surgery, Paris.

Question 2.12

What investigation has been performed? Can you identify the labelled anatomy?

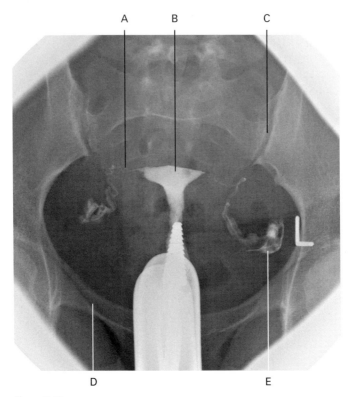

Figure 2.12

Answer
This is a hysterosalpingogram.

A: Right fallopian tube.
B: Fundus of uterus.
C: Left sacroiliac joint.
D: Right superior pubic ramus.
E: Peritoneal spill of contrast.

Don't panic, the examiner doesn't expect you to be a gynaecologist! Hysterosalpingography is predominantly used to investigate subfertility; the anatomy is well demonstrated, however, and forms only the basis for our discussion.

Clinical notes

The fallopian tubes have clinical relevance for the surgeon because they connect the uterine cavity to the peritoneal cavity. Pelvic inflammatory disease (PID) is an important mimic of a surgical abdomen in women of childbearing age.

The communication between the exterior and the peritoneal cavity is a pathway for infection for such organisms as *Neisseria gonorrhoeae*. The incidence of pelvic inflammatory disease (PID) is on the increase. Salpingitis, tubo-ovarian sepsis and endometritis often lead to lower abdominal pain, which may mimic appendicitis.

A gynaecological history is important, making note of vaginal discharge and dysuria as well as the menstrual cycle. Adnexal and cervical tenderness on vaginal examination are important signs in favour of PID. A urine dip test will often be positive for nitrites, leukocytes and erythrocytes; this does not exclude surgical disease, however. An inflamed appendix adherent to the bladder wall is a well-recognized cause of a positive urine dip test. A transabdominal pelvic or transvaginal ultrasound scan may demonstrate free fluid within the pelvis if not a primary gynaecological pathology. Referral to a gynaecologist for high vaginal swabs and commencement on appropriate antibiotics is sensible. Laparoscopy has a role if there is ongoing diagnostic uncertainty.

Question 2.13

This is a micturating cystourethrogram in a child. Can you identify the labelled anatomical regions or structures?

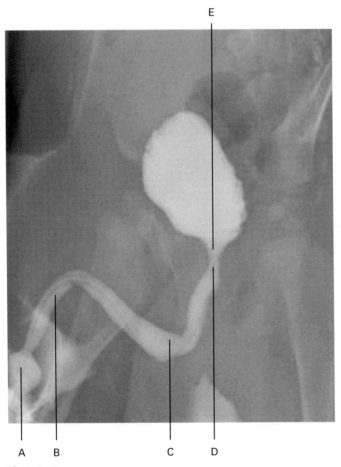

Figure 2.13

Answer

No marks for identifying the bladder.

A: Navicular fossa.
B: Penile urethra.
C: Bulbous urethra.
D: Membranous urethra.
E: Prostatic urethra.

Anatomical notes

The adult male urethra is a 20-cm long, mucous membrane lined tube, which facilitates the passage of urine from the bladder, and semen from the seminal vesicles. Urethral glands embedded within the urethral wall secrete mucus into the canal. The proximal urethra is surrounded by two muscular sphincters. The most proximal of these is the internal urethral sphincter which is composed of detrusor smooth muscle at the bladder neck and is under the control of the autonomic nervous system. The external urethral sphincter is located a short way downstream just distal to the prostate gland, at the level of the membranous urethra. It is formed from skeletal muscle and is under somatic control.

The prostatic urethra is the short segment (3–4 cm) which passes through the prostate gland between the internal and external sphincters, and is the location of the openings of the ejaculatory ducts at the verumontanum. The membranous urethra is an even shorter segment (0.5 cm) found at the level of the urogenital diaphragm and external sphincter. The remaining distal length of urethra is known as the spongy urethra and stretches from the outer edge of the urogenital diaphragm to the external urethral meatus. This portion of the urethra is surrounded by the corpus spongiosum. The spongy urethra can be subdivided into bulbous urethra, penile urethra and navicular fossa. The bulbous urethra is where the lumen temporarily widens and the openings of the bulbourethral glands of Cowper are located. Distally the urethra becomes known as the penile urethra until it reaches a further short luminal widening within the glans penis just proximal to the external urethral meatus. This portion of the urethra is known as the navicular fossa.

Clinical notes

Congenital urethral valves may occur in the proximal urethra causing obstruction to the flow of urine. Backpressure causes dilatation of the prostatic urethra, bladder and ureters and can lead to severe renal damage and occasionally failure. Most cases present either at birth or within the first few months of life. Prenatal ultrasound can often detect signs of the condition before the child is born. Treatment is to transurethrally resect the valves. Milder cases may present later on in early childhood with recurrent urinary tract infections and difficulty with micturition.

In adults a retrograde urethrogram is performed acutely for patients who are suspected to have a urethral injury secondary to trauma. Typically the patient has sustained a pelvic fracture. Blood seen at the external urethral meatus or a failed single attempt at urinary catheterization are the usual triggers for this investigation. The site of injury is typically found to be at the membranous urethra (urogenital diaphragm) where partial or complete rupture has occurred.

William Cowper (1666–1709) British surgeon and anatomist.

Question 2.14

Review the images. Identify which pelvis is male and which is female, and give three anatomical differences evident on these plain films to support your answer.

A

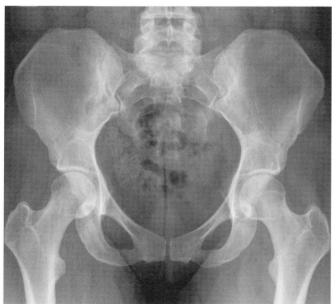

B

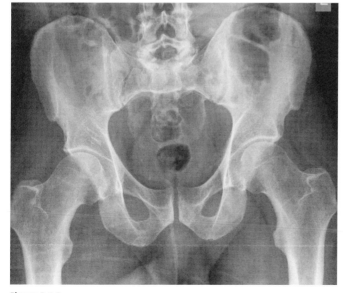

Figure 2.14

Answer

A: Female.

B: Male.

1. The pelvic inlet is wider and oval shaped in the female. In the male it is comparatively narrower and heart shaped.
2. The soft tissue shadow of the penis and scrotum is just visible at the bottom of image B.
3. The angle formed by the inferior pubic rami meeting at the symphysis is obtuse in the female and acute in the male. This is a reliable sign.

Clinical notes

There are two key morphological differences between the male and female pelvis, the first is due to the exclusive role of the female pelvis as a birth canal, necessitating a wider and shallower pelvic cavity. The second is the stronger bone structure associated with a heavier muscular build in the male.

The examiner may go on to facilitate a discussion about the anatomy of the bony and ligamentous pelvis. You will find helpful material in Chapter 4 on orthopaedics.

Question 2.15

What investigation has been performed? Can you identify the labelled anatomy?

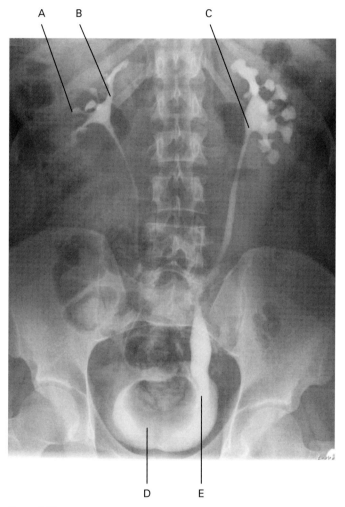

Figure 2.15

Answer

This is an intravenous urogram (IVU).

A: Renal papilla.
B: Right upper pole major calyx.
C: Left pelvi-ureteric junction (PUJ).
D: Bladder.
E: Left vesico-ureteric junction (VUJ).

Anatomical notes

The outer renal cortex contains the glomeruli and convoluted tubules, whereas the inner medulla contains the nephron loops and collecting ducts. The medulla of each kidney is typically composed of between 8 and 15 renal pyramids with apices facing the hilum. The pyramids are separated by renal columns, through which the interlobar vessels run.

The renal papillae are the apices of the renal pyramids, and can be seen as the central depressions on the contrast-filled minor calyces on an excretory phase IVU. The minor calyx is the first named portion of the macroscopic collecting system. Several minor calyces unite to form a major calyx. The major calyces unite at the renal hilum to form the renal pelvis. The renal pelvis receives urine from the calyces and drains it into the ureter for transport to the bladder.

The ureter is a 25-cm long muscular tube, which drains urine from the kidney to the bladder by way of peristalsis. Conventionally the ureter has three main anatomical regions, the abdominal, pelvic and intravesical portions. The ureter commences at the pelvi-ureteric junction and traverses in a caudal direction through the abdomen as a retroperitoneal structure just anterior to psoas major.

The right ureter lies deep to the second part of duodenum and lateral to the IVC. It is crossed anteriorly by the gonadal vessels, and the right colic and ileocolic vessels. The left ureter is also crossed anteriorly by gonadal vessels and the corresponding large bowel vessels (left colic).

The abdominal portions of the ureters end, and the pelvic portions begin, as these structures pass over the pelvic brim. This descriptive junction is anterior to the sacroiliac joints, and superficial to the point where the common iliac arteries bifurcate to form the external and internal iliacs, bilaterally. The ureters descend caudally on the corresponding lateral walls of the pelvis to a point level with the ischial spines. At this point each ureter angles medially and anteriorly to enter the bladder.

The intravesical portion of each ureter is approximately 2 cm long as the structure takes an oblique course to open into the bladder at the vesico-ureteric junction (VUJ). The ureter is said to obtain its blood supply from small branches of the numerous nearby arteries along its course.

Clinical notes

Most ureteric calculi encountered within the UK population are predominantly calcium oxalate in composition. Ureteric colic is a common and particularly painful condition managed acutely by the dedicated urologist or general surgeon. Traditionally an intravenous urogram has been the gold-standard imaging investigation to establish the diagnosis. This test has, however, been replaced by non-contrast computed tomography (NCCT); NCCT is more sensitive and also has the advantage of picking up alternative pathologies (symptomatically mimicking colic) in the absence of stone disease. The risks of contrast-related anaphylactic reaction are of course also eliminated. The price for this investigation, however, is an increase in radiation exposure to the patient, which in younger patients who are investigated for recurrent colic episodes causes concern regarding cumulative dose burden.

Despite the now questionable role of an IVU, it is superior to NCCT at displaying the collecting system anatomy, for such purposes as an MRCS viva. The ureter narrows at three distinct sites on its journey to the bladder. Each site is predisposed therefore as a location for the impaction of a migrating stone:
1. The pelvi-ureteric junction (PUJ).
2. The pelvic brim.
3. The vesico-ureteric junction (VUJ).

These sites should be reviewed especially carefully on a plain abdominal film if the diagnosis of ureteric colic is entertained. Although the traditional teaching is that 90% of renal/ureteric stones can be seen on a plain film, the recent literature suggests that 60% is a more realistic figure. Overlying bowel gas, deeper bony structures and potential false positives such as phleboliths make identification of stones very difficult. Stones composed of struvite, matrix, uric acid and xanthine are relatively radiolucent on plain film. The more calcium within a stone, the more likely it is to stand out. Stones less than 0.5 cm in size have a very high likelihood of spontaneous passage to the bladder.

3

Head and neck

Question 3.1

What does the image show and can you name the labelled structures?

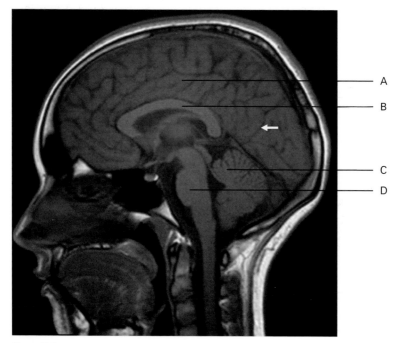

Figure 3.1

Answer
This is an MR image (T1 weighted) showing a sagittal slice through the brain.

A: Cerebral hemisphere.
B: Corpus callosum.
C: Cerebellum.
D: Pons, a component of the brainstem.

Anatomical notes

The brain can be divided into the two cerebral hemispheres and the cerebellum. The cerebellum is separated from the cerebrum by the tentorium cerebelli, an extension of dura mater.

The two cerebral hemispheres are separated by a deep cleft termed the great longitudinal fissure. Lying within this fissure is the falx cerebri, so-named from its sickle-shaped form. This is another strong fold of dura mater that is narrow anteriorly where it attaches to the crista galli of the ethmoid bone and broad posteriorly as it attaches to the tentorium cerebelli.

The cerebral hemispheres consist of a superficial layer of grey matter called the cerebral cortex. In order to maximize the surface area, the cortex is arranged into ridges (gyri) and troughs (sulci). Many sulci–gyral patterns are consistently located in individuals as to allow each hemisphere to be divided into four lobes – frontal, temporal, parietal and occipital.

The central sulcus of Rolando separates the frontal and parietal lobes. Immediately anterior to this is the precentral gyrus which houses the primary motor cortex. Immediately posterior to the central sulcus (and therefore within the parietal lobe) is the post-central gyrus, the site of the primary somatosensory cortex. A clear separation between the parietal and occipital lobes can only be seen medially as the parieto-occipital sulcus (white arrow). The occipital lobe is the site of the primary visual cortex. The temporal lobe lies below the lateral fissure of Sylvius and is further divided by three major gyri which run parallel to the Sylvian fissure – superior, middle and inferior temporal gyri. The primary auditory cortex is located within the superior temporal gyrus.

Beneath the cortex lies an extensive network of nerve fibres which can be classified into three groups:

Association fibres: connecting cortical sites within the same hemisphere.

Projection fibres: passing between the cerebral cortex and more caudal structures such as the thalami, basal ganglia and spinal cord.

Commissural fibres: passing between the two hemispheres.

The major body of commissural fibres is the corpus callosum. This acts as a bridge between the two hemispheres.

Clinical notes

Intracranial tumours can be divided into supra-tentorial (above tentorium cerebelli) or infra-tentorial (below tentorium cerebelli). Further anatomical classification is achieved by assigning findings to within the brain parenchyma (intra-axial) or between brain and dura mater (extra-axial). Most intra-axial, supra-tentorial tumours are gliomas or metastases. Most extra-axial, supra-tentorial tumours are meningiomas.

Luigi Rolando (1773–1831) Italian anatomist, University of Turin.

Franciscus Sylvius (1614–1672) Professor of Medicine, Leiden University.

Question 3.2

What does the image show and can you name the labelled structures?

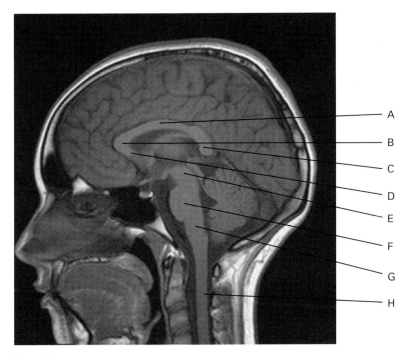

Figure 3.2

Answer

This is an MR image (T1 weighted) showing a sagittal slice through the brain.

A: Body of corpus callosum.
B: Genu of corpus callosum.
C: Splenium of corpus callosum.
D: Rostrum of corpus callosum.
E: Midbrain.
F: Pons.
G: Medulla oblongata.
H: Spinal cord.

Anatomical notes

The corpus callosum is anatomically divided into the **rostrum, genu, body** and **splenium**. The splenium connects the two occipital cortices and as such links visual function.

The brainstem is divided from cranial to caudal, into the midbrain, pons and medulla oblongata. Caudally, and at the level of the foramen magnum, the medulla becomes continuous with the spinal cord. The brainstem is also connected to the cerebellum via six groups (three on each cerebellar hemisphere) of white matter tracts, termed the superior, middle and inferior cerebellar peduncles. They connect the cerebellum to the midbrain, pons and medulla respectively.

Numerous ascending and descending fibre tracts traverse the brainstem and link the spinal cord to the cerebral hemispheres. Other fibres originate or terminate within brainstem nuclei. Probably the most well known of all the brainstem nuclei are those of the cranial nerves (III–XII). The brainstem also houses the reticular formation, a matrix of neurons and nuclei which control important functions such as consciousness, perception of pain and cardiovascular and respiratory regulation.

Question 3.3

What does the image show and can you name the labelled structures?

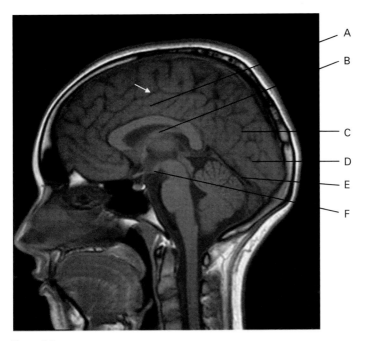

Figure 3.3

Answer

This is an MR image (T1 weighted) showing a sagittal slice through the brain.

A: Cingulate gyrus.
B: Fornix.
C: Parieto-occipital fissure.
D: Calcarine sulcus.
E: Tentorium cerebelli.
F: Mammillary body.

Anatomical notes

The calcarine sulcus lies medially within the occipital lobe and provides the location of the primary visual cortex.

The cingulate gyrus is part of the limbic system which is involved with processing, learning and memory. It also plays a role in formation of emotion. Note how the cingulate gyrus wraps around the corpus callosum and how it is limited superiorly by the cingulate sulcus (white arrow).

The fornix is a C-shaped bundle of nerve fibres that links the hippocampus (also part of the limbic system) to the mammillary body of the hypothalamus.

Question 3.4

What does the image show and can you name the labelled structures?

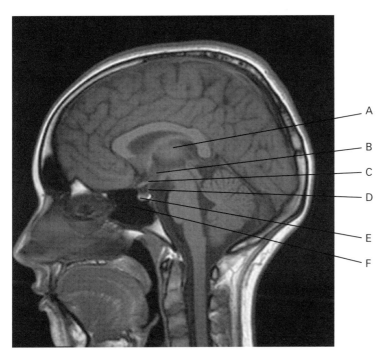

Figure 3.4

Answer

This is an MR image (T1 weighted) showing a sagittal slice through the brain.

A: Thalamus.
B: Hypothalamus.
C: Optic chiasma.
D: Infundibulum (pituitary stalk).
E: Pituitary gland.
F: Sphenoid sinus.

Anatomical notes

The two thalami lay on either side of the midline and together with the hypothalamus form the lateral walls of the third ventricle (see later images).

As the name suggests, the hypothalamus lies beneath the thalami and has strong physiological connections to the pituitary gland. The pituitary gland (hypophysis) is connected to the hypothalamus via the infundibulum (pituitary stalk) and consists of two major components, the anterior pituitary (aka adenohypophysis; glandular, not neural in origin) and the posterior pituitary (aka neurohypophysis). Under the influence of the hypothalamus the anterior pituitary releases the following hormones into the general circulation.

- Growth hormone.
- Prolactin.
- Thyroid stimulating hormone.
- Luteinizing hormone.
- Follicle stimulating hormone.
- Adrenocorticotrophic hormone.

The posterior pituitary gland is a true neuronal structure and is part of the endocrine system. It stores and releases hormones that are synthesized by the hypothalamus, such as oxytocin and vasopressin.

The pituitary gland lies within the sella turcica of the sphenoid bone. Note its relationship to the sphenoid sinus and the optic chiasma.

Clinical notes

Neurosurgeons utilize the fact that the pituitary gland lies postero-superiorly to the sphenoid sinus when excising pituitary tumours. This operation is termed a transphenoidal resection and is performed by inserting an endoscope into the nostril towards the base of the tumour.

Pituitary tumours that compress the optic chiasma may cause bitemporal hemianopia. Alternatively, pituitary tumours may cause under- or over-production of its particular hormones leading to conditions such as adrenal insufficiency or Cushing's disease (adrenocortical control), precocious puberty or hypogonadism (sexual dysfunction), diabetes insipidus (vasopressin deficiency) or gigantism/acromegaly or dwarfism (growth hormone irregularity).

Question 3.5

What does the image show and can you name the labelled structures?

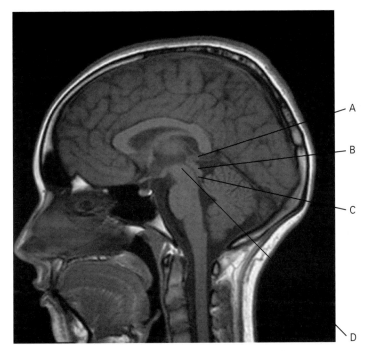

Figure 3.5a

Answer
This is an MR image (T1 weighted) showing a sagittal slice through the brain.

A: Pineal gland.
B: Tectum (quadrigeminal plate).
C: Aqueduct of Sylvius.
D: Cerebral peduncle.

Anatomical notes

The midbrain consists of the dorsal tectum and two ventral cerebral peduncles. The peduncles contain important nuclei such as those of the oculomotor and trochlear nerves and also contain numerous nerve fibres including corticospinal tracts.

The cerebral aqueduct of Sylvius runs through the midbrain, connecting the 3rd and 4th ventricles.

The tectum lies posteriorly to the cerebral aqueduct and consists of four colliculi (quadrigeminal bodies); two superior and two inferior (see Figure 3.5a). The superior colliculi are involved in visual pathways whereas the inferior colliculi form part of the auditory system.

The trochlear (4th) nerve is the only cranial nerve to emerge from the dorsal aspect of the brainstem. It originates just below the inferior colliculus and then curves around the midbrain to run anteriorly to supply the superior oblique muscle.

Ventral to the cerebral aqueduct at the level of the superior colliculus lies the oculomotor nucleus. The oculomotor nerve (3rd) has three main functions: it supplies all of the extraocular muscles except the superior oblique (trochlear) and the lateral rectus (abducens nerve); it carries parasympathetic neurones which act upon the sphincter pupillae muscle of the iris causing papillary constriction, and it innervates levator palpebrae superioris which allows elevation of the upper eyelid.

The pineal gland is situated immediately rostral to the superior colliculus. It is an endocrine organ that releases melatonin and is thought to be involved in the sleep/waking cycle.

Clinical notes

A third nerve palsy may result from either a lesion of its nucleus or from direct compression of the nerve by a lesion along its course e.g. a tumour or an aneurysm. Related to its anatomical supply this will result in (1) inability to move the eye upwards, downwards or medially, (2) dilation of the pupil and (3) ptosis.

As a hint to remember this, think about the 'fight or flight' sympathetic response. When faced with danger your eyes open wide (as a sympathetic response) – this will therefore also happen when the opposing parasympathetic supply from the oculomotor nerve is lost.

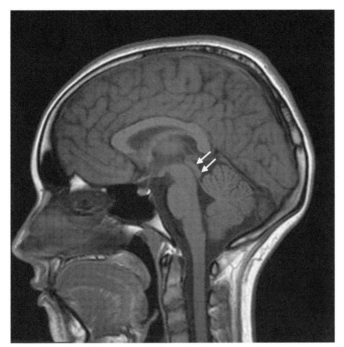

Figure 3.5b Mid-sagittal magnetic resonance image (T1 weighted) through the brain demonstrating the superior and inferior colliculi (white arrows).

Question 3.6

What does the image show and can you name the labelled structures?

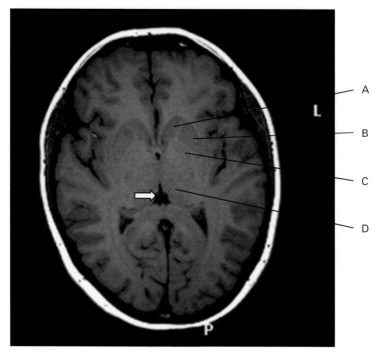

Figure 3.6

Answer

This is an MR image (FLAIR sequence – this is still a T2-weighted sequence but parameters are slightly changed to cause CSF to appear dark. This allows lesions lying in or close to the ventricles to be seen more clearly). It is an axial slice through the brain.

A: Left caudate nucleus.
B: Left putamen.
C: Left globus pallidus.
D: Left thalamus.

Anatomical notes

The caudate nucleus, globus pallidus and putamen, together with the amygdala (not shown) constitute the basal ganglia, nuclear masses lying within the deep white matter of the cerebrum.

Together the globus pallidus and putamen are called the lentiform nucleus. A further term, the corpus striatum is given to the combination of the caudate and lentiform nuclei.

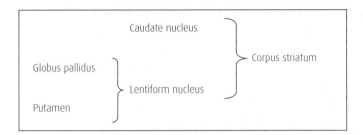

As well as being closely anatomically related, the components of the corpus striatum are also closely functionally related, being involved in the control of posture and movement. The corpus striatum also has important connections with other parts of the brain, particularly the thalamus.

The two thalami, one in each cerebral hemisphere, lie postero-medial to the lentiform nuclei. You will appreciate from Figure 3.6 that the thalami form the lateral walls of the third ventricle (white arrow). In the majority of individuals the thalami are connected across the midline by a collection of nerve fibres and nuclei termed the interthalamic adhesion or massa intermedia. The thalami contain many nuclei and play an important role in relaying information to and from various parts of the cortex.

Question 3.7

What does the image show and can you name the labelled structures?

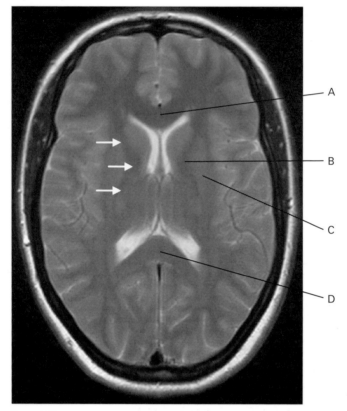

Figure 3.7a

Answer

This is an MR image (T2 weighted) showing an axial slice through the brain.

A: Rostrum of corpus callosum.
B: Left internal capsule.
C: Left lentiform nucleus.
D: Splenium of corpus callosum.

Anatomical notes

This axial image serves as a reminder that the corpus callosum consists of four parts, the anterior rostrum, genu, body and the posterior splenium. The image also illustrates the commissural nature of the corpus callosum as fibres traverse both cerebral hemispheres.

The internal capsule is divided anatomically into three parts, an anterior limb, a genu and a posterior limb (depicted as white arrows on the right internal capsule). Note its important anatomical relations – medially lies the caudate nucleus and the thalamus whilst the lentiform nucleus lies laterally.

The internal capsule consists of projection fibres which carry impulses both from and to the cerebral cortex. For further explanation let us consider a group of fibres which pass from the cortex to the spinal cord (e.g. corticospinal tracts). The neurones of these tracts originate from cell bodies in the cerebral cortex, particularly the primary motor cortex (pre-central gyrus). In order to pass to the spinal cord the axons of the neurones first traverse a massive collection of white matter fibres called the corona radiata. They then pass through the internal capsule and enter the cerebral peduncles of the midbrain. From there they traverse the brainstem and enter the cord. A greater appreciation of this can be obtained by looking at a coronal section through the brain and brain-stem. See if you can identify the labelled structures by applying the knowledge you have just learnt.

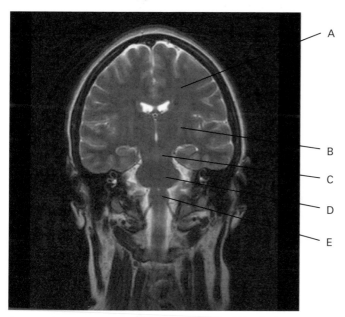

Figure 3.7b Magnetic resonance image (T2 weighted) showing a coronal slice through the brain.

A: Left corona radiata.
B: Left internal capsule.
C: Left cerebral peduncle of the midbrain.
D: Pons.
E: Medulla.

Question 3.8

What does the image show and can you name the labelled structures?

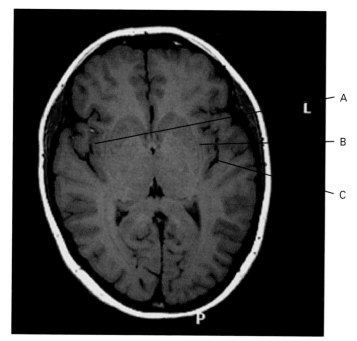

Figure 3.8a

Answer

This is an MR image (FLAIR sequence) showing an axial slice through the brain.

A: Right insula.
B: Left claustrum.
C: Left Sylvian (lateral) fissure.

Anatomical notes

You will recall that the Sylvian fissure separates the frontal and parietal lobes above from the temporal lobe below. Thus, immediately lateral to the Sylvian fissure on this image is the temporal lobe.

Deep to the Sylvian fissure is an area of cortex called the insula (Island of Reil). Its function is still under much investigation, but it is thought to be related to the limbic system and has also been linked to playing a possible role in addiction.

The claustrum is a thin sheet of grey matter whose function still remains unknown. It lies lateral to the putamen, within a body of white matter. It divides the surrounding white matter into a medially positioned external capsule and a lateral extreme capsule. The extreme capsule is therefore seen to lie between the claustrum and the insula. See the figure below for further clarification.

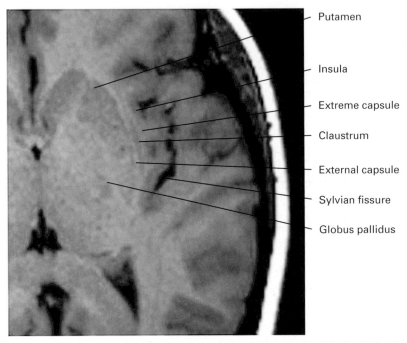

Putamen

Insula

Extreme capsule

Claustrum

External capsule

Sylvian fissure

Globus pallidus

Figure 3.8b Magnified axial (T1-weighted) magnetic resonance image of the brain, showing the left lentiform nucleus and surrounding structures.

Johann Christian Reil (1759–1813) a German physician, physiologist, anatomist and psychiatrist.

Question 3.9

What does the image show and can you name the labelled structures?

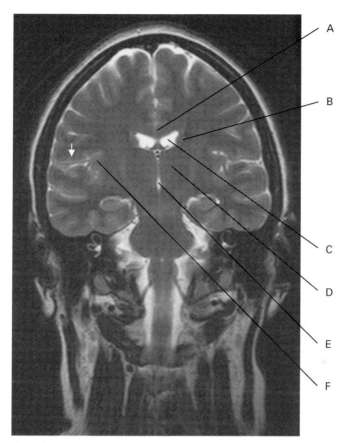

Figure 3.9

Answer

This is an MR image (T2 weighted) showing a coronal slice through the brain.

A: Corpus callosum.
B: Left caudate nucleus.
C: Left lateral ventricle.
D: Left thalamus.
E: 3rd ventricle.
F: Right insula.

Anatomical notes

This image serves to highlight important anatomical relations to the ventricular system. It can be seen that the lateral ventricles are housed by the following structures:

Roof – the corpus callosum.

Floor – in part by the superior aspect of the thalami.

Lateral walls – the caudate nuclei.

As a reminder, the lateral walls of the 3rd ventricle are formed from the medial portion of the thalami.

The insula is once again seen to be a cortical structure that lies deep to the Sylvian fissure (white arrow).

Question 3.10

What does the image show and can you name the labelled structures?

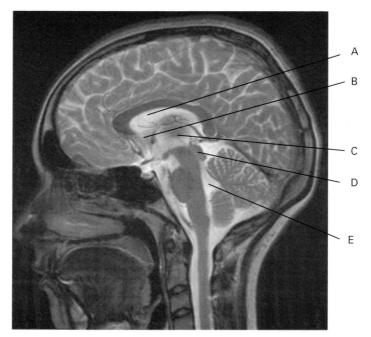

Figure 3.10

Answer

This is an MR image (T2 weighted) showing a sagittal slice through the brain.

A: Lateral ventricle.
B: Interventricular foramen of Monro.
C: 3rd ventricle.
D: Aqueduct of Sylvius.
E: 4th ventricle.

Anatomical notes

The ventricular system consists of a series of chambers that produce and circulate cerebrospinal fluid (CSF). Cerebrospinal fluid flows from the lateral ventricle to the 3rd ventricle through the interventricular foramen of Monro. The cerebral aqueduct of Sylvius connects the 3rd and 4th ventricles. Fluid exits the 4th ventricle into the subarachnoid space through lateral foramina of

Luschka (to the cerebellopontine angles) and through a central aperture called the foramen of Magendie (to the cisterna magna). The CSF then flows in the subarachnoid space and is eventually reabsorbed into venous sinuses through arachnoid granulations. These are hypertrophied invaginations of arachnoid mater that pass through the dural wall into the lumen of the sinuses.

Cerebrospinal fluid is produced by modified ependymal cells in the choroid plexus. Choroid plexus is present in all parts of the ventricular system except the aqueduct of Sylvius and the frontal and occipital horns of the lateral ventricles. Approximately 500 ml of CSF is produced per day but usually only 150 ml is found circulating at any one point. Thus CSF turnover occurs 3–4 times per day.

Clinical notes

Hydrocephalus denotes abnormal accumulation of cerebrospinal fluid within the ventricular system. It is caused by either obstruction of the flow of CSF (non-communicating) or by failure of reabsorption of the CSF (communicating).

Causes of communicating hydrocephalus include subarachnoid haemorrhage, meningitis, Chiari malformations and congenital absence of arachnoid granulations.

Obstruction may be a result of external compression or caused by an intraventricular mass lesion.

Clinical signs include those of raised intracranial pressure e.g. reduced conscious level, papilloedema and bulging fontanelles in infants.

Decompression of the dilated ventricles can be achieved by surgical insertion of a connecting shunt to either the jugular vein or more commonly the abdominal peritoneum.

Alexander Monro (secundus) (1733–1817) Scottish physician and educator. He was the son of Alexander Monro (primus) and then fathered Alexander Monro (tertius). All three were Professor of Anatomy at Edinburgh University.

Francois Magendie (1783–1855) French physiologist.

Hubert von Luschka (1820–1875) German anatomist.

Question 3.11

What does the image show and can you name the labelled structures?

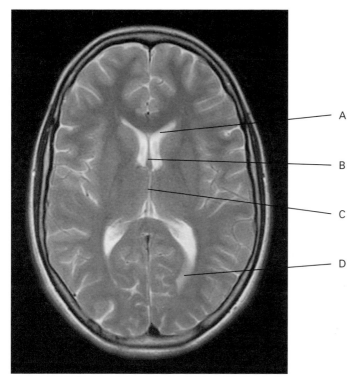

Figure 3.11a

Answer
This is an MR image (T2 weighted) showing an axial slice through the brain.

A: Frontal horn of the left lateral ventricle.
B: Septum pellucidum.
C: 3rd ventricle.
D: Occipital horn of the left lateral ventricle.

Anatomical notes

The lateral ventricles are anatomically divided based upon where their projections lie within the brain. Thus, their anterior projections are called the frontal horns, their posterior projections are called the occipital horns and their inferior projections are termed the temporal horns.

The frontal horn is also considered to be the part of the lateral ventricle that lies anterior to the foramen of Monro.

In normal brains the temporal horns are very rarely seen. They become more visible in patients with brain atrophy or in patients suffering from hydrocephalus. Indeed, a conspicuous temporal horn is often the earliest sign of developing hydrocephalus. See the figure below, a CT scan showing an axial section of the brain. The temporal horns are dilated and are seen to lie on either side of the midbrain. The white material bathing the midbrain is subarachnoid blood – the cause of the patient's hydocephalus.

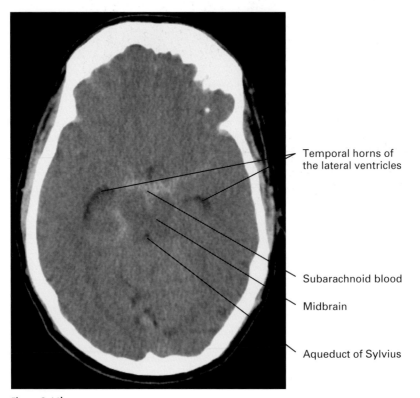

Temporal horns of
the lateral ventricles

Subarachnoid blood

Midbrain

Aqueduct of Sylvius

Figure 3.11b

The septum pellucidum forms the medial wall of the frontal horns of the lateral ventricles. It is a thin membranous sheet that extends in a sagittal plane from the corpus callosum above to the fornix below.

Question 3.12

What does the image show and can you name the labelled structures?

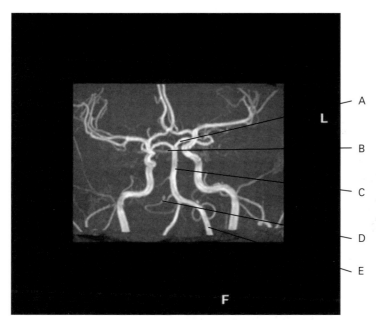

Figure 3.12

Answer
This is an MR image (MIP) demonstrating the arterial supply to the brain – the circle of Willis.

A: Left posterior cerebral artery.
B: Right superior cerebellar artery.
C: Basilar artery.
D: Right anterior inferior cerebellar artery.
E: Left vertebral artery.

Anatomical notes

The blood supply to the brain comes from anterior and posterior circulations which are connected via communicating branches. The posterior circulation constitutes the convergence of the two vertebral arteries to form the basilar artery. This occurs at the ponto-medullary junction. The basilar artery then runs the length of the pons over its ventral surface to eventually terminate by bifurcation into the right and left posterior cerebral arteries. The posterior cerebral arteries curve around the midbrain to supply the occipital lobes and the inferomedial aspect of the temporal lobe.

The vertebral and basilar arteries give off many important branches which supply blood to the cerebellum, brainstem and spinal cord. At their distal ends the vertebral arteries give rise to the posterior inferior cerebellar arteries (supplying the inferior aspect of the cerebellum) and the anterior and posterior spinal arteries (supplying the medulla and spinal cord). At its proximal end the basilar artery gives rise to the anterior inferior cerebellar arteries which, as their name suggests, supply the anterior and inferior aspect of the cerebellum. The basilar artery also provides blood supply to the pons by way of numerous pontine branches and to the inner ear via the labyrinthine arteries. Just before its terminal bifurcation into the posterior cerebral arteries, the basilar artery gives rise to the paired superior cerebellar arteries which again, as their name suggests, supply the superior aspect of the cerebellum.

Clinical notes

The circle of Willis is a common site for cerebral aneurysms. Their spontaneous rupture can lead to subarachnoid haemorrhage. Angiography used to be the primary procedure to characterize the aneurysm, however, this is being replaced by computer tomography angiography (CT angiograms) whereby 3D reconstruction is available. Treatment can be conservative, radiological intervention or surgical. Surgery, involving craniotomy and the placement of a metal clip across the neck of the aneurysm is becoming superseded by vascular intervention where small coils, particles or glue are implanted into the aneurysm to cause haemostasis and prevent further leakage of blood.

Thomas Willis (1621–1675). English physician and Oxford Professor.

Question 3.13

What does the image show and can you name the labelled structures?

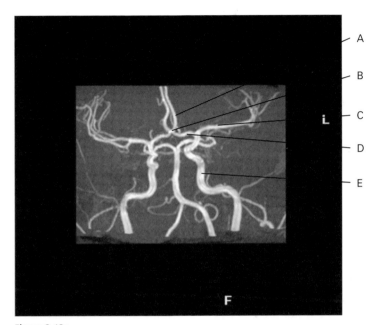

Figure 3.13a

Answer

This is an MR image (MIP) demonstrating the arterial supply to the brain – the circle of Willis.

A: Left anterior cerebral artery (A2).
B: Anterior communicating artery.
C: Left middle cerebral artery.
D: Left anterior cerebral artery (A1).
E: Left internal carotid artery.

Anatomical notes

This image has been used to highlight the anterior cerebral circulation which contributes to the circle of Willis.

The anterior circulation is formed from the internal carotid arteries. These arteries terminate by forming the anterior and middle cerebral arteries. This bifurcation occurs just lateral to the optic chiasma.

The middle cerebral artery is larger than the anterior or posterior cerebral arteries. From its origin it passes laterally to enter the Sylvian fissure. Here, it subdivides into branches that supply the inner cortices of the lateral fissure such as the auditory cortex and the insula and into other branches which course laterally to supply most of the lateral cortical surface of the brain. Please note that the reason for using the term 'most' in the previous sentence is because the anterior cerebral artery supplies a strip of lateral cortex which lies within about 2.5 cm of the great longitudinal fissure (See figure below).

You may recall the cortical homunculus, a visual representation of the 'body within the brain'. This displays bodily parts sprawled over the primary motor cortex. In this representation the leg sits adjacent to the great longitudinal fissure and as a result is supplied by the anterior cerebral artery, whilst the remainder of the body is positioned over the lateral surface of the cortex and as such is served by the middle cerebral artery.

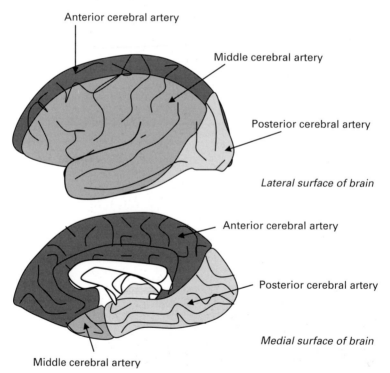

Figure 3.13b Distribution of blood supply over the cortex.

The anterior cerebral artery courses antero-superiorly above the optic nerve to lie between the two frontal lobes within the great longitudinal fissure. At this point the two anterior cerebral arteries are linked by the small anterior communicating artery. After a short anterior course the anterior cerebral artery then passes postero-superiorly over the corpus callosum to supply the medial surface of the frontal and parietal lobes (see Figures 3.13b, d).

Neurosurgeons divide the anterior cerebral artery into two sections to allow a more accurate description of where lesions such as aneurysms may occur. The A1 section occurs from the origin of the anterior cerebral artery to where it meets the anterior communicating artery. After this point the anterior cerebral artery is referred to as A2.

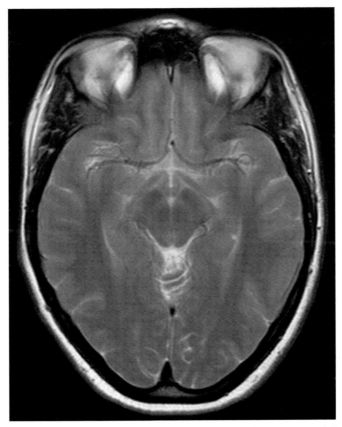

Figure 3.13c T2-weighted magnetic resonance image showing an axial slice through the brain at the level of the midbrain (note the ventral cerebral peduncles and the dorsal superior colliculi).

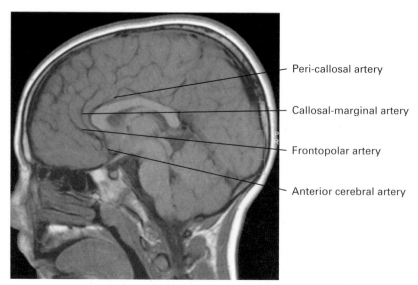

Peri-callosal artery

Callosal-marginal artery

Frontopolar artery

Anterior cerebral artery

Figure 3.13d T1-weighted magnetic resonance image showing an almost midsagittal slice through the brain. Note how the anterior cerebral artery (A2) courses superiorly over the corpus callosum and whilst doing so it gives rise to certain branches. It is highly unlikely that you will be expected to name the branches of the anterior cerebral artery but if you can then you're sure to pick up top marks! The most anterior branch, coursing towards the frontal pole, is aptly named the frontopolar artery. The branch that lies over the superior surface of the corpus callosum is called the peri-callosal artery, while the other branch which traverses over the cingulate gyrus is termed the callosal-marginal artery.

Question 3.14

What does the image show and can you name the labelled structures?

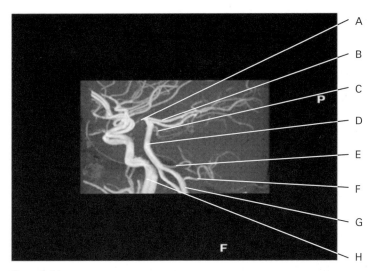

Figure 3.14

Answer

This is an MR image (MIP) in sagittal-oblique section demonstrating the arterial supply to the brain – the circle of Willis.

A: Posterior communicating artery.
B: Posterior cerebral artery.
C: Superior cerebellar artery.
D: Basilar artery.
E: Anterior inferior cerebellar artery.
F: Posterior inferior cerebellar artery.
G: Vertebral artery.
H: Internal carotid artery.

Anatomical notes

This sagittal-oblique image of the circle of Willis demonstrates the separate anterior and posterior circulations. It also reveals the posterior communicating artery linking the posterior cerebral and internal carotid arteries, thus completing the circle of Willis. (It can be fairly minuscule!)

Remember: if you are ever faced with a similar image just apply basic principles and look for what you know. You will recognize the two vertebral arteries combining to form the basilar artery. Follow the basilar to its termination and you will find the posterior cerebral arteries.

Question 3.15

What does the image show and can you name the labelled structures?

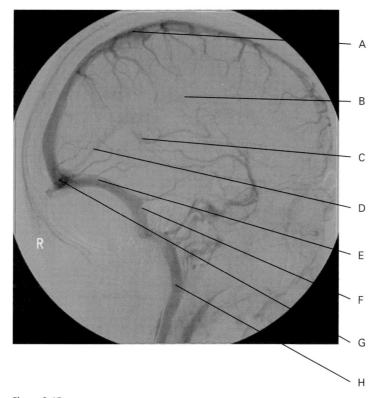

Figure 3.15a

Answer

This is a cerebral venogram showing the venous drainage of the brain in sagittal section.

A: Superior sagittal sinus.
B: Inferior sagittal sinus.
C: Great cerebral vein of Galen.
D: Straight sinus.
E: Transverse sinus.
F: Sagittal sinus.
G: Confluence of sinuses.
H: Internal jugular vein.

Anatomical notes

The veins of the brain are termed sinuses. They contain no valves and run independent of the arteries. They exist within the separated layers of dura mater – dura mater consists of two layers – a superficial layer constituting the cranium's periostium and a deeper layer, the dura mater proper.

The superior and inferior sagittal sinuses run in the upper and lower borders of the falx cerebri respectively. The superior sagittal sinus drains into the confluence of sinuses, located at the internal occipital protuberance. Blood then passes predominantly into the right transverse sinus. Blood in the inferior sagittal sinus combines with blood in the great cerebral vein of Galen to form the straight sinus. This in turn drains predominantly into the left transverse sinus. Transverse sinuses become continuous with sigmoid sinuses which in turn deliver blood to the internal jugular veins. See Figure 3.15b for an oblique view.

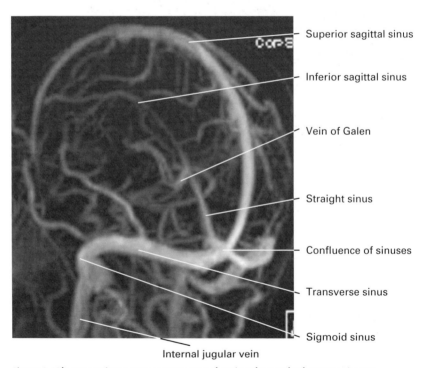

Figure 3.15b Magnetic resonance venogram showing the cerebral venous sinuses.

Galen (approximately 120–207 AD). Physician to the School of Gladiators and to the Roman Emperor Marcus Aurelius.

Question 3.16

What does the image show and can you name the labelled structures?

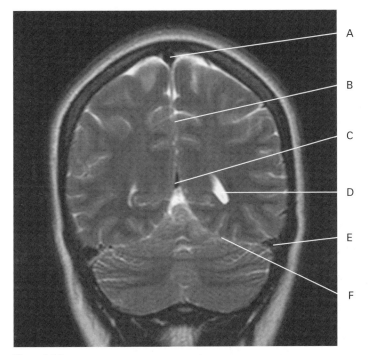

Figure 3.16

Answer
This is an MR image (T2 weighted) showing a coronal section through the brain
and cerebellum.

A: Superior sagittal sinus.
B: Falx cerebri.
C: Straight sinus.
D: Occipital horn of the left lateral ventricle.
E: Lateral aspect of the left transverse sinus.
F: Tentorium cerebelli.

Anatomical notes

This image has been used to further highlight the positions of the venous sinuses.
    The key to this image is identifying the cerebellum. Once you have achieved
this you can identify the overlying tentorium cerebelli, and because the

cerebellum is visualized you will know that you are dealing with posterior cranial structures such as the occipital horns of the lateral ventricles and the straight and transverse sinuses.

Also note the position of the falx cerebri lying within the great longitudinal fissure with the superior sagittal sinus running along its superior margin.

Clinical notes

Intracranial haemorrhage may be intra-cerebral (within the substance of the brain) or extra-cerebral. Intra-cerebral haemorrhage may occur spontaneously (e.g. from severe hypertension or from an underlying arteriovenous malformation (AVM)), or secondary due to trauma (penetrating or blunt) or an underlying tumour.

Extra-cerebral haemorrhages can be classified according to their position amongst the meningeal layers. Subarachnoid haemorrhage (SAH) is a bleed within the subarachnoid space (i.e. the space between the arachnoid and pia mater) and can occur spontaneously or as a result of trauma. The majority of spontaneous SAHs occur from the rupture of cerebral aneurysms. Other spontaneous causes include bleeding from an AVM or from a tumour.

Subdural haemorrhage is the result of tears within the veins that bridge the subdural space (i.e. the space between the dura and arachnoid mater). Trauma is by far the most common cause either from a fall or as a result of sheering forces (as in sudden acceleration-deceleration injuries such as in road traffic accidents or shaken-baby syndrome). The elderly and alcoholics are particularly susceptible because brain atrophy increases the length of the bridging veins and makes them more likely to tear. Subdural haemorrhages often present late as a result of the relatively slow accumulation of blood. This is in contrast to extradural haematomas which present relatively early as they result from arterial haemorrhage.

Extradural (also known as epidural) haemorrhage is usually traumatic, the classic scenario being a blow to the side of the head causing injury to the middle meningeal artery. There is almost always an associated cranial fracture. The result is an expansile haematoma which lies between the dura mater and the cranium. As the cranium can not expand the brain bears the force. As a result, extradural haematomas require urgent surgical intervention to prevent pressure coning and death.

Question 3.17

What does the image show and can you name the labelled structures?

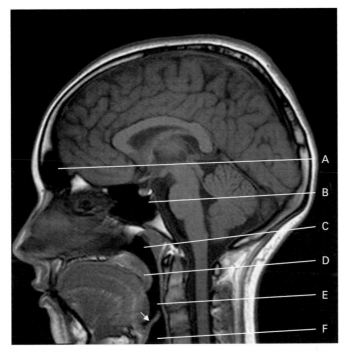

Figure 3.17

Answer

This is an MR image (T1 weighted) showing a sagittal slice through the brain.

A: Frontal sinus.
B: Sphenoid sinus.
C: Nasopharynx
D: Soft palate with uvula.
E: Oropharynx.
F: Laryngopharynx.

Anatomical notes

Paranasal sinuses are air-filled spaces within facial bones that communicate with the nasal cavity. They are named according to the bones in which they lie: frontal, maxillary (aka Antrum of Highmore), ethmoid and sphenoid. The ethmoidal sinus is described as having anterior, posterior and middle compartments. Paranasal sinuses are thought to have many functions, including reducing the weight of the skull, increasing the resonance of the voice and heating and humidifying inspired air.

The pharynx is a fibromuscular tube which forms the upper part of the alimentary canal. It extends from the base of the skull to the cricoid cartilage and over its course it becomes the posterior relation to the nasal, oral and laryngeal cavities. On this basis it is divided into three parts:

1. **Nasopharynx** – from the base of the skull to the upper border of the soft palate at the level of C1 vertebra. It contains the opening of the auditory tube.
2. **Oropharynx** – from the lower surface of the soft palate to the upper border of the epiglottis (short white arrow in Figure 3.17, approximately C3).
3. **Laryngopharynx** – from the upper border of the epiglottis to the level of the cricoid cartilage (C6). Here it becomes continuous with the oesophagus.

The pharynx has mucosal, submucosal and muscular layers. The muscular layer is formed by five paired muscles, the superior, middle and inferior constrictors and the stylopharyngeus and palatopharyngeus muscles. The constrictors form an outer circular coat by combining posteriorly in the midline to form a raphé whilst the stylopharyngeus and palatopharyngeus muscles contribute by forming an inner longitudinal layer. The stylopharyngeus is innervated by the IXth cranial nerve, glossopharyngeal, whereas the other pharyngeal muscles are all innervated by the vagus nerve (specifically by branches from the pharyngeal plexus and by branches from the recurrent laryngeal nerve).

Clinical notes

The inferior constrictor muscle is actually composed of two parts, a superior thyropharyngeal and an inferior cricopharyngeal, named after the laryngeal cartilages from which they attach. Posteriorly, between these two muscle groups is a potentially weak area known as Killian's dehiscence. It is through this space that a pharyngeal pouch (also known as Zenker's diverticulum) may protrude.

Individuals with a pharyngeal pouch may be asymptomatic but more commonly they present with dysphagia, a sense of having a lump in the neck, regurgitation of food or halitosis. It rarely causes pain.

Diagnosis can be made through barium swallow or endoscopy.

Treatment varies depending on its size. Often small, asymptomatic pouches (i.e. those discovered incidentally) require no further intervention. The current preferred treatment option for larger, symptomatic pouches is to close the defect by way of fibreoptic endoscopic stapling.

Nathaniel Highmore (1613–1685). English surgeon and anatomist, studied in Oxford and worked most of his life in Sherborne, Dorset.

Gustav Killian (1860–1921). German laryngologist.

Friedrick Albert von Zenker (1825–1898). German pathologist and physician, celebrated for his discovery of trichinosis (parasitic disease).

Question 3.18

What does the image show and can you name the labelled structures?

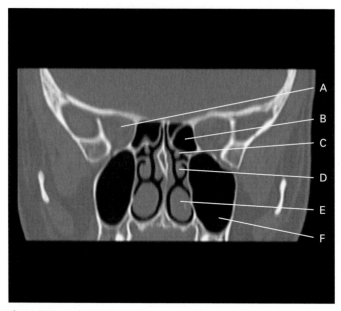

Figure 3.18

Answer

This is a CT scan showing the paranasal sinuses in coronal plane.

A: Right orbit.
B: Left ethmoidal sinus.
C: Left superior turbinate.
D: Left middle turbinate.
E: Left inferior turbinate.
F: Left maxillary sinus (antrum).

Anatomical notes

Turbinates (also known as conchae) are bony shelves surrounded by erectile soft tissue. There are three on each side named according to their position in the nasal cavity. They cover their corresponding meati (recesses) into which the paranasal sinuses drain:

- **Sphenoid sinus** – drains into the spheno-ethmoidal recesses (posterior to the sphenoid sinus and superior to the superior turbinate).

- **Posterior ethmoidal sinus** – drains into the superior meatus (inferior to the superior turbinate).
- **Anterior and middle ethmoidal** plus the **frontal** and **maxillary sinuses** drain into the middle meatus (inferior to the middle turbinate).
- **Nasal lacrimal gland** drains into the inferior meatus (below the inferior turbinate).

Thus, all the sinuses except the sphenoid and posterior ethmoidal sinuses drain into the middle meatus.

Clinical notes

Individuals suffering from sinusitis have the potential for the infection to spread into the cranium either directly or indirectly. Causes of direct spread include trauma, surgery and chronic bone infections such as osteomyelitis, leading to the necrotic breakdown of sinus walls. Trauma resulting in an open skull fracture allows organisms to seed directly into the brain and raises the potential for abscess formation. In the same way, surgery also carries this risk!

Indirect extension tends to occur through haematogenous spread. Connecting the vasculature of the sinus mucosa and the venous sinuses of the brain is a valveless venous network. This network provides a potential route for bacteria to enter the cranium from the sinuses.

Thrombophlebitis originating in the veins of the sinus mucosa can migrate through the emissary veins of the skull, the dural venous sinuses, the subdural veins and into the cerebral veins. This type of indirect extension can cause selective infection of the subdural space leading to a subdural empyema.

Question 3.19

What does the image show and can you name the labelled structures?

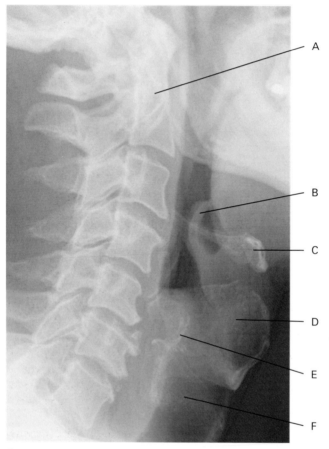

Figure 3.19

Answer
This is a lateral radiograph of the cervical spine.

A: Odontoid peg.
B: Epiglottis.
C: Hyoid bone.
D: Thyroid cartilage.
E: Arytenoid cartilage.
F: Cricoid cartilage.

Anatomical notes

The larynx forms the upper part of the lower respiratory tract and lies from approximately C3 to C6.

It consists of a cartilaginous skeleton which is suspended from the hyoid bone above to the trachea below by membranes and ligaments.

The cartilages can be divided into:
- Three large unpaired cartilages – thyroid, cricoid and epiglottis.
- Three smaller paired cartilages – arytenoid, corniculate and cuneiform.

The thyroid cartilage is the largest of the laryngeal cartilages and sits between the hyoid bone above and the cricoid cartilage below. It consists of two lamina (left and right) which join anteriorly in the midline to form a superior projection termed the laryngeal prominence or 'Adam's apple'. The posterior margins of the thyroid lamina do not fuse. Instead both posterior margins elongate to form superior and inferior horns. The inferior horns articulate with the cricoid cartilage whilst the superior horns attach to the hyoid bone via lateral thyrohyoid ligaments.

The epiglottis is a leaf-shaped cartilage that attaches to the posterior aspect of the thyroid cartilage just below the laryngeal prominence. It projects posterosuperiorly with its superior margin lying above the level of the hyoid bone.

The cricoid cartilage forms a complete circle but is shaped more like a signet ring as it has a much broader posterior aspect (the lamina) than its narrow anterior arch. The posterior lamina possesses two articular facets on each side – one laterally for articulation with the inferior horn of the thyroid cartilage and one superiorly for articulation with the arytenoid cartilage.

The paired arytenoid cartilages are pyramid-shaped consisting of a base, an apex, a medial surface and an antero-lateral surface. The base of each cartilage sits upon the superior aspect of lamina of the cricoid cartilage, whilst the apices articulate with the corniculate cartilages. The cuneiform cartilages lie anterior to the corniculate cartilages.

The laryngeal ligaments can be divided into extrinsic and intrinsic ligaments. Extrinsic ligaments include:
- **Thyrohyoid membrane** – running between the hyoid bone above and the thyroid cartilage below. The posterior edges of the thyrohyoid membrane are thickened and form the lateral thyrohyoid ligaments. This thickening also occurs anteriorly forming the median thyrohyoid ligament.
- **Cricotracheal ligament** – linking the cricoid cartilage above to the trachea below.
- **Hyo-epiglottic ligament** – linking the antero-superior border of the epiglottis to the posterior aspect of the hyoid bone.

Intrinsic ligaments include:
- **Cricothyroid ligament** – inferiorly this is attached to the arch of the cricoid cartilage. Superiorly it is fixed at two points – anteriorly to the thyroid

cartilage and posteriorly to the arytenoid cartilages. Between the two fixation points the cricothyroid ligament is devoid of further attachment. Thus, it has a free superior border. This border is thickened to form the vocal ligament, which is under the 'true' vocal cord.

- **Quadrangular membrane** – on either side, this runs from the lateral margins of the epiglottis to the anterolateral surface of the arytenoid cartilage. It has both free upper and lower margins. The free lower margin lies above the vocal ligaments and is thickened to form the vestibular ligament under the vestibular fold (also known as the false vocal cord). The free upper borders of the quadrangular membrane are also thickened to form the aryepiglottic folds.

The presence of the vestibular folds and the vocal folds allows the larynx to be divided into three main regions:

1. An upper chamber called the vestibule which lies between the laryngeal inlet and the vestibular folds.
2. A middle chamber, lying between the vestibular folds and the vocal folds.
3. A lower chamber, termed the infraglottic space, which lies between the vocal folds and the laryngo-tracheal junction.

Intrinsic muscles act upon the various components of the larynx in order to satisfy particular functions. For example, they facilitate the closure of the laryngeal inlet by manipulating the epiglottis in order to prevent food boluses entering the lower respiratory tract. They also alternate the tension applied to the vocal cords in order to allow phonation. All intrinsic muscles of the larynx are innervated by the recurrent laryngeal nerve except the cricothyroid muscles which are innervated by the superior laryngeal nerves. Both recurrent and superior laryngeal nerves are branches of the vagus nerve (X).

Clinical notes

In emergency situations when the airway is blocked above the level of the vocal folds the cricothyroid membrane can be punctured to establish an airway. In the emergency room this can be achieved by making a 2 cm incision through the cricothyroid membrane using a scalpel and then widening the hole by rotating the scalpel or by using a clamp. A size 6 or 7 endotracheal tube can then be inserted and its cuff inflated. Ventilation can then be provided by attaching the tube to an oxygen source. The full name for this procedure is a cricothyrotomy.

Question 3.20

What does the image show and can you name the labelled structures?

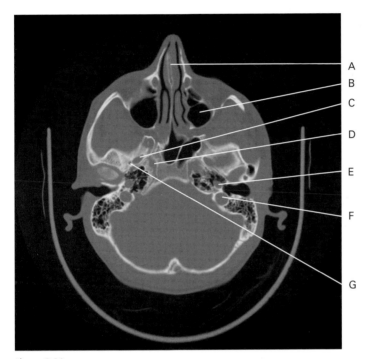

Figure 3.20

Answer
This is a CT image showing an axial slice through the base of the skull.

A: Nasal septum.
B: Left maxillary sinus (antrum).
C: Right foramen ovale.
D: Right foramen lacerum.
E: Left carotid canal.
F: Left jugular foramen.
G: Right foramen spinosum.

Anatomical notes

The foramen ovale is situated in the medial aspect of the body of the sphenoid bone. It transmits the mandibular branch of the trigeminal nerve, the accessory meningeal artery and emissary veins from the middle cranial fossa to the infratemporal fossa.

Just postero-lateral to the foramen ovale is the foramen spinosum. Through this passes the middle meningeal artery and vein and the recurrent branch of the mandibular nerve.

The foramen lacerum exists between the sphenoid and temporal bones and is formed by superior and inferior defects in the carotid canal. It is covered by fibro-cartilage and as such it is not a true foramen. The nerve of the pterygoid canal (Vidian nerve) forms in the cartilaginous substance of the foramen lacerum and travels forward with the corresponding artery towards the anterior cranial fossa. Emissary veins are likely to be the only true structures that traverse the foramen lacerum. The internal carotid artery rests on the fibro-cartilage but does not pierce it.

The carotid canal forms where the petrous apex articulates with the sphenoid and occipital bones. It transmits the internal carotid artery and the carotid plexus of nerves.

The jugular foramen is located behind the carotid canal and is formed in front by the petrous temporal bone and behind by the occipital bone. It is divided into three compartments:

Anterior compartment – transmits the inferior petrosal sinus.

Middle compartment – transmits the IXth, Xth and accessory nerves.

Posterior compartment – transmits the sigmoid sinus (becoming the internal jugular vein) and the meningeal branches from the occipital and ascending pharyngeal arteries.

Clinical notes

Base of skull fractures represent a significant injury. Characteristic signs include blood in the paranasal sinuses, cerebrospinal fluid otorrhea, raccoon eyes (peri-orbital bruising) and Battle's sign (mastoid ecchymosis).

Vidus Vidius (1508–1569). Italian surgeon, anatomist and physician.

Question 3.21

What does the image show and can you name the labelled structures?

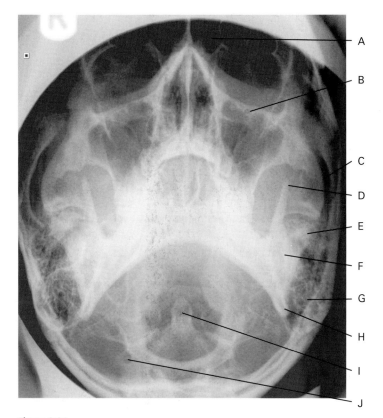

Figure 3.21

Answer
This is a plain radiograph of the facial bones.

A: Ethmoid air cells.
B: Infra-orbital foramen.
C: Zygomatic arch.
D: Coronoid process of mandible.
E: Head (condyloid process) of mandible.
F: Ramus of mandible.
G: Mastoid air cells.
H: Angle of mandible.

I: Dens.
J: Foramen transversarium.
  - What muscle attaches to D?
  - What nerve passes through B?
  - What passes through J?
  - What muscle originates from C?
  - What muscle attaches to the lateral surface of F?
  - What muscle attaches to the medial surface of H?
  - What structures run in the mandibular canal?
  - What foramen lies in the body of the mandible?
  - What ligaments do you know that connect the dens to the occiput?
  - What movements occur at the atlanto-occipital and atlanto-axial joints?

Anatomical notes

The zygomatic arch is formed by the zygomatic process of the temporal bone and the temporal process of the zygomatic bone. The masseter muscle takes its origin here and passes inferiorly to insert into the lateral side of the ramus of the mandible. The ramus of the mandible continues posteriorly as the neck and head and anteriorly as the coronoid process. Temporalis attaches to the latter whilst the lateral pterygoid muscle inserts into the pterygoid fovea (a hollow in the medial surface of the neck of the mandible).

The mandibular foramen lies on the medial surface of the ramus of the mandible, lipped anteriorly by a small tongue-like bony protrusion called the lingula. The inferior alveolar nerve (a branch of the mandibular division of the trigeminal nerve) and vessels pass through the foramen and run infero-medially in the mandibular canal. The inferior alveolar nerve gives rise to the mental nerve which passes through the mental foramen in the body of the mandible to supply the skin and mucous membrane of the lower lip and labial gum.

The medial pterygoid muscle attaches to the medial surface of the angle of the mandible. The medial and lateral pterygoids plus the masseter and temporalis constitute the muscles of mastication. These muscles are all innervated by the trigeminal nerve.

The dens (odontoid process or peg) is a projection of bone passing superiorly from the anterior portion of C2 (or axis). It articulates anteriorly with a facet found on the posterior surface of the anterior arch of C1 (atlas). Numerous ligaments connect the dens to the occiput:

- The **transverse ligament** runs across the back of the dens attaching to the lateral margins of C1. **Longitudinal fibres** run from the posterior part of the body of C2 to attach to the basiocciput. The fibres of the transverse and longitudinal ligaments cross and are thus collectively termed the **cruciform ligament**.

- Linking the apex of the dens to the anterior margin of the foramen magnum is the **apical ligament**.
- Attaching to dens, on either side of the apical ligment, are the paired **alar ligaments**. These run obliquely to the lateral margins of the foramen magnum.
- The **tectorial membrane** is a continuation of the posterior longitudinal ligament (ligament running the length of the spine on the posterior surface of the vertebral bodies). It is attached to the posterior surface of the body of C2 and runs superiorly to the anterior margin of the foramen magnum.

Extension, lateral and forward flexion of the head occurs at the atlanto-occipital joint and rotation occurs at the atlanto-axial joint. No rotation is possible at the atlanto-occipital joint.

4

Orthopaedics

Question 4.1

Name the labelled structures on this pelvic radiograph.
Use the radiograph to describe the joints and ligaments that give stability to the pelvis.

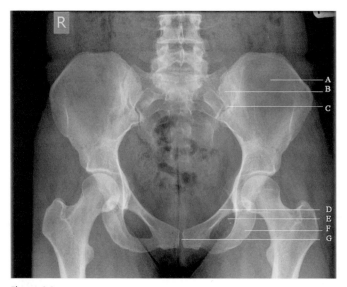

Figure 4.1

Answer
A: Ilium.
B: Sacrum.
C: Sacroiliac joint.

D: Iliopectineal line.
E: Obturator foramen.
F: Ishium.
G: Pubic symphysis.

Anatomical notes

The pelvis is made up from the os innominatum, the sacrum and the coccyx, bound to each other by dense ligaments. The joints of the pelvis include the lumbosacral, sacrococcygeal and sacroiliac joints and the pubic symphysis.

The sacroiliac joints are strong, weight-bearing synovial joints between the articular surfaces of the sacrum and ilium. There is some interlocking of the bones between the irregular surface elevations and depressions which helps decrease their mobility and allows the transfer of body weight to the hips. The sacrum is suspended between the iliac bones and is firmly attached to them by interosseous and posterior sacroiliac ligaments. The sacrotuberous and sacro-spinous ligaments allow only limited movement at the inferior end of the sacrum which allows resilience when the vertebral column needs to withstand increased loading.

- **Sacrotuberous ligament**: passes from ischial tuberosity to the side of sacrum and coccyx.
- **Sacrospinous ligament**: passes from the ischial spine to the side of sacrum and coccyx.

These two ligaments help define two important exits from the pelvis:

- **Greater sciatic foramen**: formed by greater sciatic notch and sacrospinous ligament.
- **Lesser sciatic foramen**: formed by lesser sciatic notch and sacrotuberous ligament.

The sacrum is made up of five fused vertebrae and is roughly triangular in shape. The anterior border of its upper part is termed the sacral promontory. Its anterior aspect presents a central mass, a row of four anterior sacral foramina on each side (transmitting the upper four sacral anterior rami) and, lateral to these, the lateral masses of the sacrum. The superior aspect of the lateral mass on each side forms a fan-shaped surface termed the ala.

Posteriorly, lies the sacral canal, continuing the vertebral canal, bounded by short pedicles, strong laminae and diminutive spinous processes. Perforating through from the sacral canal is a row of four posterior sacral foramina on each side. Inferiorly, the canal terminates in the sacral hiatus, which transmits the 5th sacral nerve.

Question 4.2

Name the structures labelled on the hip radiograph.
Use the plain film to describe the attachments of the capsule and ligaments which provide strength to the hip joint.
What is the anatomy of the blood supply to the femoral head? What is the significance of this in relation to the management of a fractured neck of femur?

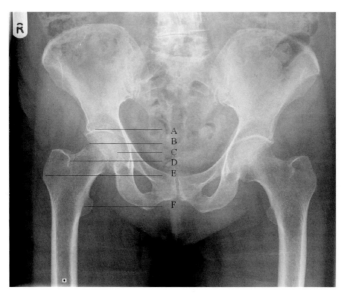

Figure 4.2

Answer
A: Acetabular roof.
B: Posterior acetabular rim.
C: Fovea.
D: Intertrochanteric crest.
E: Greater trochanter.
F: Lesser trochanter.

Anatomical notes

The hip joint is a synovial ball-and-socket joint between the hemispherical head of the femur and the acetabulum of the inominate bone. The acetabulum has a central depression known as the acetabular fossa, surrounded by a horse-shoe-shaped articular surface, which is deficient inferiorly as the acetabular notch.

The cavity of the acetabulum is deepened by the acetabular labrum, which is known as the transverse acetabular ligament where it crosses the acetabular notch. The capsule of the hip joint attaches to the acetabular labrum and passes to the intertrochanteric line of the femur anteriorly. Posteriorly, it attaches to the neck of the femur above the intertrochanteric crest. The capsule is re-inforced by three ligaments:

- Iliofemoral ligament (Y-shaped).
- Pubofemoral ligament (triangular).
- Ischiofemoral (spiral-shaped).

The blood supply to the hip joint is derived from:

- Obturator artery.
- Medial and lateral circumflex femoral arteries.
- Nutrient artery of the femur.

From the intertrochanteric ridge, some fibres of the joint capsule retinacula are reflected back up the neck to the head of femur. The retinacula blood vessels, derived principally from the medial and lateral circumflex femoral vessels, lie within these fibres and provide the main blood supply to the adult head of femur. Disruption of the retinacular vessels can render the head of femur avascular.

Clinical notes

The simplest classification of fractured neck of femur is into extracapsular and intracapsular fractures. Fifty per cent of fractured neck of femurs are intracapsular and at risk of avascular necrosis of the femoral head, secondarily to disruption of the blood supply.

Management differs according to the type of fracture. The majority of intracapsular fractures are treated by hemiarthroplasty due to the risk of subsequent avascular necrosis of the femoral head. Extracapsular fractures can be stabilized with a dynamic hip screw (DHS) as replacement of the femoral head is not indicated.

Question 4.3

What type of images are these?
Name the labelled structures.
What is compartment syndrome? Describe the clinical symptoms.

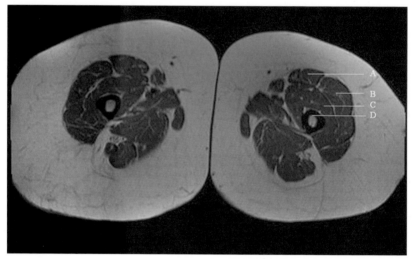

Figure 4.3

Answer

These are axial T1-weighted images through both thighs – illustrating the muscles within each of the compartments.

Some of the anterior compartment structures have been labelled.

A: Rectus femoris.
B: Vastus lateralis.
C: Vastus intermedialis.
D: Femoral shaft.

Anatomical notes

The thigh is divided into anterior, medial and posterior compartments by septae passing from the femur to deep fascia of the thigh, the fascia lata. The latter has the following attachments:

- Posteriorly: sacrum, coccyx, sacrotuberous ligament and ischial tuberosity.
- Laterally and posteriorly: iliac crest.
- Superiorly: inguinal ligament, pubic arch, pubic tubercle and body of pubis.
- Distally: exposed bony parts of the knee and is continuous with the crural fascia.

The muscles of the anterior thigh include:

- Psoas.
- Iliacus.
- Tensor fascia latae.
- Sartorius.
- Quadriceps femoris.

With the exception of tensor fascia latae (superior gluteal nerve), the muscles are supplied by the femoral nerve.

Clinical notes

Compartment syndrome can occur when swelling occurs in a compartment secondary to oedema, inflammation or haematoma. This initially impedes venous flow, but further increase in compartment pressure prevents inflow of oxygenated blood and can lead to muscle ischaemia and ultimately necrosis.

Causes:

- Crush injuries.
- Prolonged limb compression eg. tight POP, prolonged surgery.
- Open/closed fractures.
- Reperfusion injury.

Clinical signs and symptoms:

- Pain out of proportion to injury sustained.
- Pain on passive stretching of the affected muscle.
- Muscle tenderness.
- Sensory loss.
- Weakness.

Treatment depends on the cause of the compartment syndrome, although the basic principle remains the same: release of pressure. If required, removal/splitting of plaster immobilization and bandaging should be performed. Compartment pressures can be measured – if elevated or there is strong clinical suspicion, fascitomies must be performed. Decreased pulses and sensation are late clinical signs and treatment should not be delayed due to their absence.

Question 4.4

Name the structures on this axial MR scan.
Which level has the scan been taken at?
Explain the Trendelenburg test.

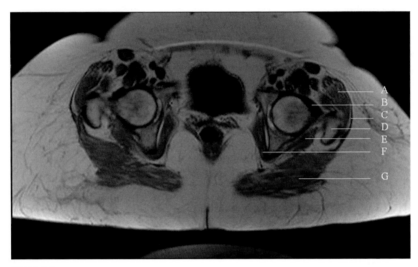

Figure 4.4

Answer
This is an axial MR scan taken at the level of the hip joint.

A: Tensor fascia lata.
B: Iliofemoral ligament.
C: Iliotibial tract.
D: Greater trochanter.
E: Superior gemellus.
F: Obturator internus.
G: Gluteus maximus.

Anatomical notes

The muscles of the gluteal region are separated into two groups:
- Glutei (maximus, medius and minimus).
- Deep lateral rotators (piriformis, gemilli, obturator internus and quadrates femoris).

The glutei extend and abduct the hip. Gluteus medius and minimus attach to the lateral and anterior surfaces of the greater trochanter and are supplied by the superior gluteal nerve. This nerve also supplies the tensor fascia latae in the anterior compartment and damage to it would give rise to a Trendelenburg gait (see below).

The upper quarter of the fibres of gluteus maximus insert into the gluteal tuberosity of the femur and the lower three-quarters insert into the iliotibial tract. The inferior gluteal nerve supplies gluteus maximus.

Three gluteal bursae separate gluteus maximus from the following under-lying structures.

- Trochanteric bursa: lateral side of the greater trochanter of the femur.
- Gluteofemoral bursa: superior part of the proximal attachment of vastus lateralis.
- Ischial bursa: ischial tuberosity.

Clinical notes

The Trendelenburg test is performed by asking the patient to stand on one leg. This tests the abductors of the supporting leg (gluteus medius, minimus and tensor fascia lata) which would normally pull on the pelvis causing it to tilt (and the opposite side of the pelvis to rise) to bring the centre of gravity over the supporting foot.

Reasons for a positive test:
- Gluteal paralysis.
- Gluteal inhibition.
- Coxa vara.
- Congenital dislocation of the hip.

Friedrich Trendelenburg (1844–1924). German surgeon.

Question 4.5

What imaging has been performed?
Name the labelled structures.

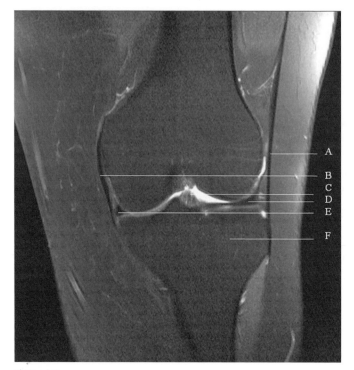

Figure 4.5

Answer
This is a coronal T1-weighted MR scan of the knee.

A: Iliotibial tract.
B: Medial collateral ligament.
C: Anterior cruciate ligament.
D: Lateral meniscus.
E: Medial meniscus.
F: Lateral tibial condyle.

Anatomical notes

The fibrous capsule of the knee joint is a cylinder of fibrous tissue between the femur and tibia, and includes the ligamentum patellae and medial collateral

ligament, but not the lateral collateral ligament. It does not completely seal the knee joint and has two major openings:
- Suprapatellar bursa (anteriorly).
- Passage of popliteus tendon (posteriorly).

The ligaments of the knee joint can be divided into extracapsular and intracapsular.

Extracapsular ligaments

- Ligamentum patellae.
- Lateral collateral ligament (LCL).
- Medial collateral ligament (MCL).
- Oblique popliteal ligament.

The two cruciate ligaments join the femoral condyles to the intercondylar ridge of the tibia within the articular capsule of the joint but outside the synovial cavity.

- **Anterior cruciate ligament (ACL):** Runs from the anterior part of the intercondylar ridge to the medial aspect of the lateral femoral condyle.
- **Posterior cruciate ligament (PCL):** Runs from the posterior part of the intercondylar ridge to the lateral aspect of the medial condyle of the tibia.

Clinical notes

In the position of 90° of flexion, the ACL and PCL are slack and can be tested by draw tests.
- **ACL**: this is the weaker of the two cruciate ligaments. It is slack when the knee is flexed and taut when fully extended, therefore preventing posterior displacement of the femur on the tibia and hyperextension of the knee joint. It is clinically tested by the **anterior draw test**.
- **PCL**: this is the stronger of the two ligaments and tightens during flexion of the knee joint, therefore preventing anterior displacement of the femur on the tibia and hyperflexion of the knee. In the weight-bearing flexed knee the PCL stabilizes the femur e.g. when walking downhill. It is clinically tested by the **posterior draw test**.

Question 4.6

What radiological investigation has been performed?
Name the labelled structures.
Describe the extensor mechanism and structures that prevent the patella from dislocating.

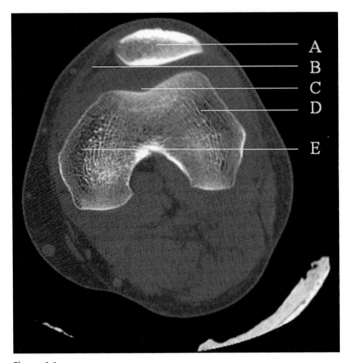

Figure 4.6

Answer
Axial CT of the left knee.

A: Patella.
B: Patella tendon.
C: Trochlea notch.
D: Lateral femoral condyle.
E: Medial femoral condyle.

Anatomical notes

The knee joint is a synovial joint between the femoral and tibial condyles, and is classified as a hinge joint. However, lateral and medial rotation can occur when the joint is flexed and medial rotation occurs during full extension. The fibula is not involved in the joint and is not a weight-bearing bone.

The patella is a sesmoid bone which lies anterior to the distal end of the femur, where it articulates posteriorly with the condyles of the femur. It is held within the extensor mechanism which arises from the quadriceps tendon and inserts onto the tibial tuberosity. The four parts of the quadriceps femoris unite to form the quadriceps tendon which attaches to the patella. The patella ligament attaches the patella to the tibial tuberosity and is the continuation of the quadriceps tendon. The patella holds the quadriceps tendon away from the distal end of the femur and increases its power and leverage.

Due to the normal valgus position of the knee, the patella is most commonly dislocated laterally. However, this is prevented by the anterior projection of the lateral femoral condyle and the medial pull of vastus medialis on the patella.

Question 4.7

Name the labelled structures on this knee radiograph.
What are the boundaries of the popliteal fossa?
What structures lie in the popliteal fossa?

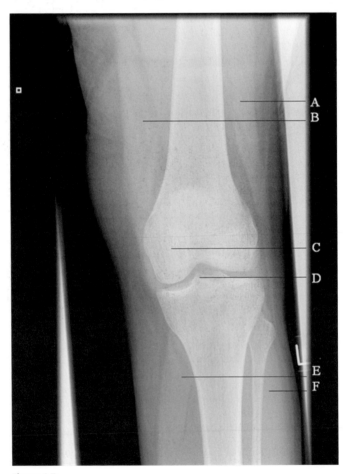

Figure 4.7

Answer

A: Biceps femoris.
B: Semimembranosus.
C: Medial femoral condyle.
D: Medial tibial spine.
E: Medial head of gastrocneumius.
F: Lateral head of gastrocneumius.

Anatomical notes

The popliteal fossa is a direct continuation of the adductor canal and has the following boundaries:
- Superolaterally: biceps femoris.
- Superomedially: semimembranosus reinforced by semitendinosus.
- Inferomedially and inferolaterally: medial and lateral heads of gastrocneumius.
- Roof: deep fascia.
- Floor: popliteal surface of femur, posterior aspect of knee joint and popliteus muscle.

The popliteal fossa contains the popliteal artery and vein. The common per-oneal nerve passes out of the fossa along the medial border of the biceps tendon; the tibial nerve is initally lateral to the popliteal vessels and then crosses over to lie medially.

The fossa also contains fat and popliteal lymph nodes.

Clinical notes

The popliteal fossa is often a site of masses which can originate from any of the contents of the fossa. An example is a Baker's cyst, located in the popliteal or gastrocneumius-semimembranosus bursae, which communicates with the posterior joint capsule. It is most commonly caused by arthritis or ligamentous tears.

William Morrant Baker (1839–1896). English surgeon, assistant to Sir James Paget for some years. Later anatomist at St Bartholomew's Hospital.

Question 4.8

Name the labelled structures on this ankle radiograph.
Describe the anatomy of the ligamentous complex around the ankle.

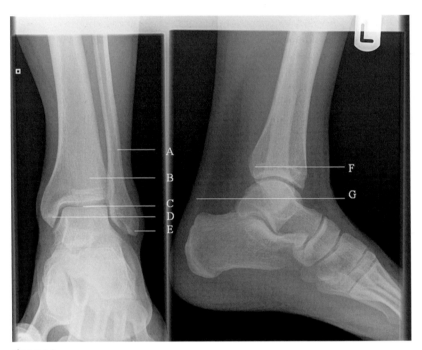

Figure 4.8

Answer
A: Fibula.
B: Tibia.
C: Talar dome.
D: Medial malleolus.
E: Lateral malleolus.
F: Posterior malleolus.
G: Achilles tendon.

Anatomical notes

The ankle joint is a synovial hinge joint between the tibia, fibula and talus. The movements which occur at this joint are dorsiflexion and plantar flexion. Inversion and eversion occur at the subtalar joint between talus and calcaneum.

There are three groups of ligaments around the ankle joint:
- Deltoid ligament.
- Lateral collateral ligamentous complex.
- Syndesmosis.

The deltoid ligament consists of a deep part, between the medial malleolus of the tibia and talus, and a superficial part which is weaker and stretched from the medial malleolus and talus, calcaneus and navicular.

The lateral collateral ligamentous complex consists of three bands:
- Anterior and posterior talofibular ligaments.
- Calcaneofibular ligament.

The syndesmosis is perhaps the most significant ligamentous complex in maintaining normal alignment of the ankle joint. It consists of four parts:
- Anterior inferior talofibular ligament.
- Posterior inferior talofibular ligament.
- Inferior transverse talofibular ligament.
- Interosseous ligament.

Question 4.9

Label the anatomical structures identified on this foot radiograph.

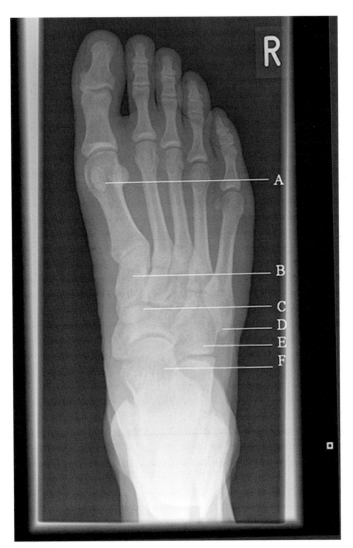

Figure 4.9

Answer
A: Head of 1st metatarsal.
B: Medial cuneiform.
C: Navicular.
D: Base of 5th metatarsal.
E: Cuboid.
F: Talus.

Anatomical notes

There are 26 bones in the foot, excluding sesmoid bones. The bones are arranged in longitudinal and transverse arches which are designed as shock absorbers to support the weight of the body and adapt to surface and weight changes.

There are three arches of the foot: two longitudinal and one transverse.

The medial arch is thought to be the strongest and consists of:

- Calcaneous.
- Talus.
- Three cuneiforms.
- Medial three metatarsals.

The lateral arch is made up of the:

- Calcaneus.
- Talus.
- Cuboid.
- Lateral two metatarsals.

The transverse arch contains:

- Cuneiforms.
- Metatarsals.
- Cuboid.

The arches are supported by the shape of the bones, by the muscles and ligaments (long and short plantar ligaments) and by the plantar aponeurosis. This results in the standing weight being taken on the calcaneus and metatarsal heads, and the arches help in giving spring to the foot in the take-off stage of walking.

Question 4.10

Label the bony anatomical structures which make up the shoulder joint. Which structures strengthen the shoulder joint?

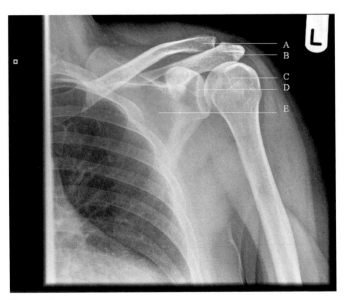

Figure 4.10

Answer
A: Clavicle.
B: Acromium.
C: Head of humerus.
D: Glenoid.
E: Scapula.

Anatomical notes

The shoulder joint is a ball-and-socket synovial joint which is highly mobile but unstable. The head of the humerus forms one third of a sphere and articulates with the glenoid cavity of the scapula. The glenoid itself is shallow, but is deepened by the glenoid labrum, a ring of fibrocartilage which encircles the glenoid cavity.

The fibrous capsule surrounds the joint and attaches medially to the margin of the glenoid and laterally to the anatomical neck of the humerus. The synovial membrane lining the capsule forms a sheath for the biceps tendon.

The capsule is strengthened by the:
- Glenohumeral ligaments.
- Coracohumeral ligaments.
- Transverse humeral ligament.

The coracohumeral ligament extends from the coracoid process to the anatomical neck of the humerus, and prevents inferior dislocation of the adducted humerus. It is only tight in adduction and provides little stability in abduction.

Clinical notes

Due to the instability of the shoulder it is commonly dislocated due to direct or indirect trauma. Anterior dislocation is commonest and is caused by excessive extension and lateral rotation of the humerus. The head of the humerus moves anteriorly and the fibrous capsule and glenoid labrum are stripped from the anterior aspect of the glenoid.

Question 4.11

Name the anatomical parts of the scapula demonstrated on this radiograph.

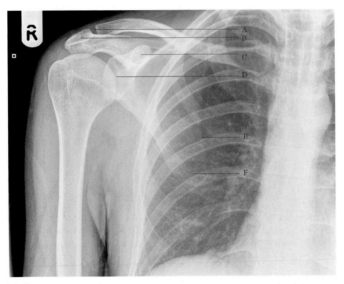

Figure 4.11

Answer
A: Acromioclavicular joint.
B: Acromion.
C: Coracoid process.
D: Glenoid.
E: Lateral border of scapula.
F: Inferior angle of scapula.

Anatomical notes

The inferior angle of the scapula overlies the 7th rib and is an important anatomical landmark.

Both the sternoclavicular and acromioclavicular joints are synovial and contain intraarticular discs. The disc of the sternoclavicular joint, together with the coracoclavicular ligament, provides vital support to the pectoral girdle by preventing medial rotation of the clavicle.

The scapula is attached to the trunk by six muscles:

● Anteriorly: pectoralis minor and serratus anterior.
● Posteriorly: trapezius, levator scapulae and rhomboids major and minor.

Serratus anterior and subscapularis separate it from the trunk. The middle fibres of trapezius assist the rhomboids in retracting the scapula, but the upper and lower fibres of trapezius assist the lower fibres of serratus anterior in lateral rotation of the scapula. The other movements are summarized below.

- Elevation: levator scapulae.
- Depression: pectoralis minor.
- Protraction: serratus anterior.
- Retraction: rhomboids.

All movements of the scapula reposition the orientation of the glenoid fossa and increase the range of movement of the arm. Pectoralis major does not attach to the scapula but inserts directly into the humerus.

Clinical notes

Serratus anterior is innervated by the long thoracic nerve of Bell (C5, C6, C7). Damage to this nerve may lead to winging of the scapula. This is demonstrated most prominently when the patient pushes their outstretched arm against a wall.

Damage to the nerve is usually secondary to either blunt or penetrating trauma. Blunt trauma classically occurs with sports injuries, e.g. from a blow to the ribs underneath an outstretched arm. Penetrating trauma may occur through surgery for breast cancer, specifically when axillary lymph node excision is performed.

Sir Charles Bell (1774–1842). Scottish anatomist, surgeon, and physiologist.

Question 4.12

Name the structures demonstrated on this axial MR of the shoulder.
Name the components of the rotator cuff.

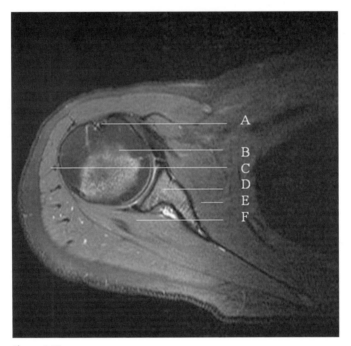

Figure 4.12

Answer
A: Long head of biceps.
B: Head of humerus.
C: Deltoid.
D: Glenoid fossa of scapula.
E: Subscapularis.
F: Infraspinatus.

Anatomical notes

The muscles of the rotator cuff act as a support to the shoulder joint by creating
an incomplete ring around it. It is made up from:
● Supraspinatus (superiorly).
● Subscapularis (anteriorly).

- Infraspinatus (posteriorly).
- Teres minor (posteriorly).

Supraspinatus, infraspinatus and teres minor attach to the facets of the greater tuberosity whereas subscapularis attaches to the lesser tuberosity. All except supraspinatus act as rotators of the arm.

Supraspinatus has the greatest practical importance. It passes over the apex of the shoulder beneath the acromium process and coracoacromial ligament, from which it is separated by the subacromial bursa. The bursa continues beneath deltoid as the subdeltoid bursa forming the largest bursa in the body.

Abduction of the shoulder is initiated by supraspinatus; deltoid can then abduct to 90°. Further movement to 180° (elevation) is brought about by rotation of the scapula upwards by trapezius and serratus anterior. Shoulder movements occur as smooth and swift actions. As soon as abduction commences at the shoulder joint, rotation of the scapula begins.

Clinical notes

Supraspinatus initiates abduction of the humerus on the scapula. If the tendon is torn, active initiation of abduction becomes impossible.

Inflammation of the supraspinatus tendon (tendinitis) is characterized by a painful arc of shoulder movement between 60–120°.

Question 4.13

Name the anatomical landmarks of the humerus.

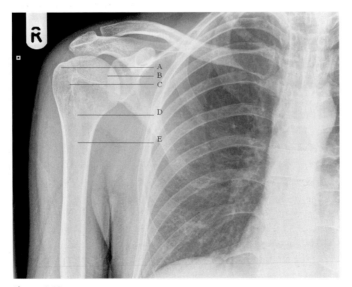

Figure 4.13

Answer
A: Greater tuberosity.
B: Head of humerus.
C: Bicipital groove.
D: Surgical neck.
E: Humeral shaft.

Anatomical notes

The humerus articulates with the scapula at the shoulder joint and the radius and ulna at the elbow joint. The head of humerus consists of one third of a sphere and faces postero-superomedially. The lesser and greater tuberosities are separated by the intertubercular (bicipital) groove, through which runs the long head of biceps.

The anatomical neck separates the head from the tuberosities. The surgical neck lies distal to the tuberosities and is where the humerus narrows to become the shaft. The axillary nerve and circumflex vessels lie here and can be damaged in a fracture to the surgical neck.

The shaft itself is circular in the section above and flattened in its lower part. It has two prominent features:

- Deltoid tuberosity.
- Spiral groove: demarcates the origin of the medial and lateral head of triceps, between which winds the radial nerve and profunda vessels.

The lower end of the humerus bears the rounded capitulum laterally for articulation with the radial head, and the spoon-shaped trochlea medially, articulating with the trochlear notch of the ulna. The medial and lateral epicondyles, on either side, are extracapsular; the medial is the larger of the two, extends more distally and bears a groove on its posterior aspect for the ulnar nerve.

Clinical notes

The humerus is a common site for fractures. The following structures are at risk in humeral fractures:

- **Surgical neck**: axillary nerve and circumflex humeral vessels.
- **Spiral groove**: radial nerve and profunda brachii.
- **Posterior aspect of medial epicondyle**: ulnar nerve.

Question 4.14

Name the labelled structures.
Which views have been taken?

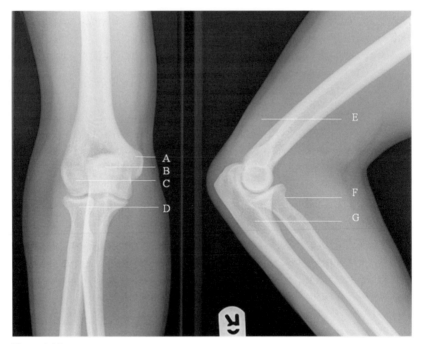

Figure 4.14

Answer
AP and lateral elbow radiographs.

A: Medial epicondyle.
B: Olecranon.
C: Lateral epicondyle.
D: Radial head.
E: Triceps.
F: Radial neck.
G: Ulna.

Anatomical notes

The elbow joint is a single synovial joint with three articulations within the same capsule:

- Humero-ulnar joint: between trochlea of humerus and trochlear notch of the ulnar (hinge joint).
- Humero-radial joint: between capitulum of the humerus and head of radius (ball-and-socket joint).
- Proximal radio-ulnar joint: between radial head and the ulnar (pivot joint).

The fibrous capsule surrounds the joint and is lined by a synovial membrane which is continuous inferiorly with the synovial membrane of the proximal radio-ulnar joint. The joint is weak anteriorly and posteriorly (allowing flexion and extension), but is strengthened medially and laterally by collateral ligaments and an annular ligament around the radial head. The fan-like radial collateral ligament extends from the lateral condyle to the annular ligament of the radius. The ulnar collateral ligament passes from the medial epicondyle to the coronoid process and olecranon.

Clinical notes

Pre-school children are vulnerable to subluxation of the radial head; known as a 'pulled elbow'. This occurs when the child is lifted by the upper limb when the forearm is pronated e.g. lifting a child up onto a bus. The sudden force tears the annular ligament and the radial head moves distally and partially out of the torn ligament.

Question 4.15

What imaging is shown below?
Name the labelled carpal bones.
Describe the boundaries of the carpal tunnel and the structures which pass through it.
What symptoms occur in carpal tunnel syndrome?

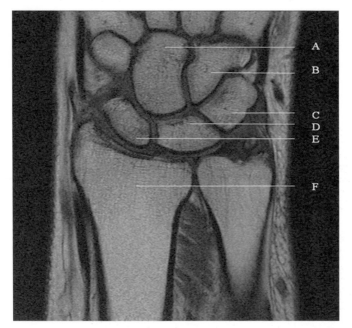

Figure 4.15a

Answer
This is a coronal MR image of the wrist.

A: Capitate.
B: Hamate.
C: Triquetrum.
D: Lunate.
E: Scaphoid.
F: Radius.

Anatomical notes

The carpal bones sit in two rows: a proximal row (triquetral, lunate, scaphoid) and a distal row (hamate, capitate, trapezoid and trapezium). The pisiform bone lies over the triquetral and is a sesmoid bone which lies in the tendon of flexor carpi ulnaris.

At the wrist, the flexor retinaculum runs transversely over underlying tendons to form a fibrous tunnel known as the carpal tunnel (see Figure 4.15b) The flexor retinaculum extends from the pisiform and hook of hamate medially to the tubercle of the scaphoid and trapezium laterally.

The carpal tunnel contains:
- Flexor digitorum profundus.
- Flexor digitorum superficialis.
- Flexor pollicis longus.
- Median nerve.

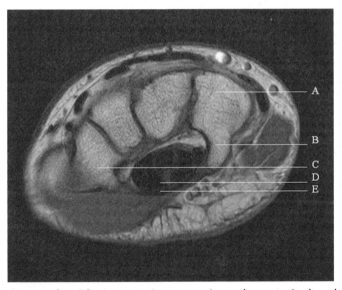

Figure 4.15b Axial wrist magnetic resonance image demonstrating boundaries and contents of carpal tunnel. A, Hamate; B, Hook of hamate; C, Trapezium; D, Flexor tendons; E, Flexor retinaculum.

Clinical notes

Carpal tunnel syndrome is compression and ischaemia of the median nerve in the carpal tunnel deep to the flexor retinaculum. It commonly affects women (females:males 8:1) aged 30–60 years.

Carpal tunnel syndrome can be caused by: pregnancy, obesity, occupation, trauma, myxoedema, rheumatoid arthritis, acromegaly, diabetes, or may be idiopathic.

A patient may present with the following symptoms:

- Pain and paraesthesia in the distribution of the median nerve in the hand – symptoms more pronounced at night.
- Wasting in thenar eminence muscles.
- Pain relieved by hanging arm out of bed and shaking it.

Question 4.16

Name the bony landmarks illustrated on the forearm radiograph.
Which features help you distinguish between the radius and ulna?

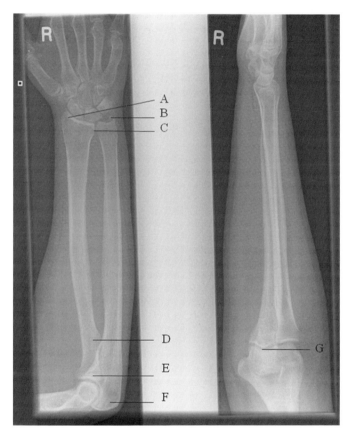

Figure 4.16

Answer
A: Radial styloid.
B: Ulna styloid.
C: Distal radio-ulnar joint.
D: Radial tubercle.
E: Radial head.
F: Olecranon.
G: Trochlea.

Anatomical notes

The radius is the shorter of the two forearm bones. Proximally it has a disc-like head, which is concave and articulates with the capitulum of the humerus. The radial neck is short and is identified as the constriction distal to the head. Just distal to this lies the tuberosity which separates the proximal end of the radius from the shaft. The distal end of the radius has an ulnar notch medially, styloid process laterally and a dorsal tubercle.

The ulna is longer and lies medially to the radius (when in anatomical position). Proximally the olecranon lies posteriorly and the coronoid process anteriorly. The trochlear notch lies on the anterior surface of the olecranon and articulates with the trochlea of the humerus. The coronoid process lies lateral to the radial notch, and inferior to this is the ulnar tuberosity. The ulnar shaft is initially thick, but narrows distally where there is a large rounded head and a small conical styloid process.

The radius and ulna are joined by an interosseous membrane. During pronation and supination, the radial shaft rotates around a relatively fixed ulnar shaft. The head of the radius rotates against the ulnar radial notch, whilst the distal radius rotates around the head of the ulna.

Clinical notes

The forearm is a common site for fractures. One of the bones may fracture in isolation or an injury, such as a fall on an outstretched hand, can cause damage to both.

The radius is subject to axial rotation due to insertion of pronator teres midway along the radial shaft. Fractures that occur proximal to this insertion will result in supination of the proximal fragment (due to the action of an unopposed biceps brachii) whilst the distal fragment will be pronated.

When fractures occur distal to the insertion of pronator teres, the actions of biceps and pronator teres are equalized.

Question 4.17

Name the bony and soft tissue structures on the hand radiograph.
Using the plain radiograph, describe the attachments of FDS and FDP and their functions.
Describe the zones of the hand, in relation to flexor tendon injury.

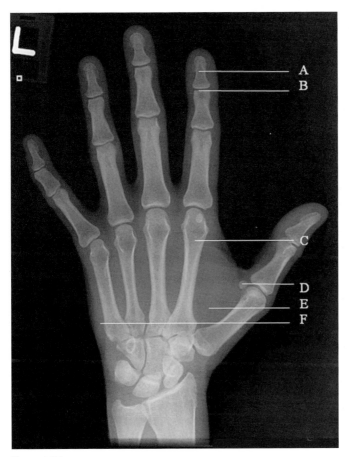

Figure 4.17

Answer
A: Distal phalanx of the left index finger.
B: Distal interphalangeal joint of the left index finger.
C: Metacarpal of the left index finger.
D: Sesmoid bone.
E: Thenar eminence.
F: Hypothenar eminence.

Anatomical notes

The long flexors of the fingers are:
- **Flexor digitorum profundus (FDP)**: inserts onto the base of the four distal phalanges and causes flexion at the distal interphalangeal joints.
- **Flexor digitorum superficialis (FDS)**: inserts into the sides of the four middle phalanges and causes flexion at the proximal interphalangeal joints.

The tendons of FDP and FDS enter the common flexor sheath deep to the flexor retinaculum and enter the central compartment of the hand before fanning into their respective digital synovial sheaths. At the base of the proximal phalanx, the tendon of FDS splits and surrounds the tendon of FDP. The FDS tendons attach to the margins of the middle phalanx and the tendons of FDP attach to the base of the distal phalanx.

The hand is divided into the following zones:

Zone 1:   Between DIP and PIPJ creases distal to insertion of FDS. This contains FDP tendon within distal sheath.

Zone 2:   Between distal palmar crease and mid-point of middle phalanx. This corresponds to the proximal part of the tendon sheath, A1 pulley, and extends to the FDS insertion containing FDS and FDP tendons.

Zone 3:   Between distal margin of carpal tunnel and distal palmar crease; contains both FDS and FDP tendons but are unsheathed.

Zone 4:   Area of carpal tunnel – contains both FDS and FDP tendons.

Zone 5:   Wrist and forearm up to carpal tunnel.

Question 4.18

What investigation has been performed?
Which level is this vertebra from?
Name the labelled structures.

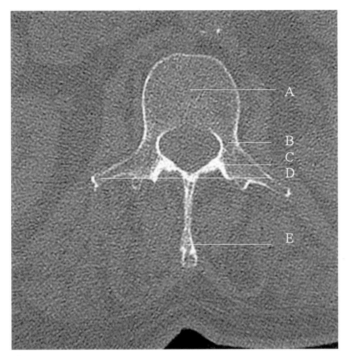

Figure 4.18

Answer
This is an axial CT of a lumbar vertebra.

The lumbar vertebrae are the largest and have strong, square, horizontal spines and have articular facets which lie in the sagittal plane.

A: Vertebral body.
B: Pedicle.
C: Lamina.
D: Transverse process.
E: Spinous process.

Anatomical notes

The spinal column is made up of 33 vertebrae. The basic vertebral structure comprises of a body and a neural arch that surrounds the vertebral canal. The neural arch is made up from a pedicle on either side, each of which support a lamina which meets posteriorly in the midline. The pedicle bears a notch above and below which, with its neighbour, forms the intervertebral foramen. The arch bears the posterior spine, lateral transverse processes and upper and lower articular facets.

The intervertebral foramina transmit the segmental spinal nerves. C1–C7 pass over the superior aspect of their corresponding cervical vertebrae, C8 passes through the foramen between C7 and T1. All subsequent nerves pass between their corresponding numbered vertebrae and the one below.

Clinical notes

Each vertebra ossifies from three primary centres, one for each side of the arch and one for the body. Occasionally the body develops from two centres and failure of one of these to form results in formation of a hemivertebra, leading to a congenital scoliosis. Spina bifida results from failure of the two arch centres to fuse posteriorly, and particularly occurs in the lumbar region. Usually this is not associated with any neurological abnormality (spina bifida occulta). Rarely, there is a gross defect of one or several arches with protrusion of the spinal cord or its coverings.

Question 4.19

What type of image is shown here?
Name the labelled structures.

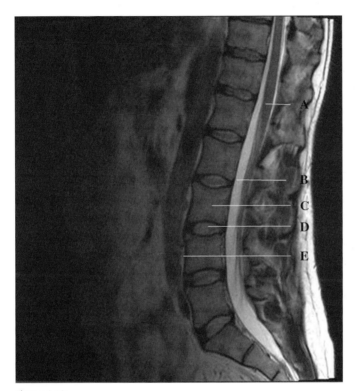

Figure 4.19

Answer

This is a T2-weighted sagittal lumbar spine MR scan.

A: Spinal cord (conus medullaris).
B: Cerebrospinal fluid.
C: Vertebral body.
D: Intervertebral disc.
E: Anterior longitudinal ligament.

Anatomical notes

The vertebral bodies are supported from occiput to sacrum by continuous anterior and posterior longitudinal ligaments. The anterior longitudinal ligament is wide, strong and firmly attached to both vertebral bodies and discs, whereas the posterior longitudinal ligament is narrower, weaker and attached firmly only to the intervertebral discs. The longitudinal ligaments continue superiorly as the anterior and posterior atlanto-occipital membranes to attach to the foramen magnum.

Three ligaments join the vertebral arches: the supraspinous ligament (between tips of the spines), the interspinous ligaments (between the spines) and the ligamentum flavum (between laminae). The supraspinous and interspinous ligaments are thickened above C7 to form the ligamentum nuchae which attaches to the external occipital protuberance.

At least one quarter of the vertebral column's length is due to the intervertebral discs. They possess a fibrous outer annulus fibrosus and an inner nucleus pulposus which consists of cartilage/collagen/water semi-fluid gel.

Clinical notes

The nucleus pulposus lies slightly posteriorly and becomes dehydrated with age. The comparatively thin posterior part of the annulus fibrosus may rupture allowing the nucleus pulposus to herniate posteriorly into the vertebral canal. This most commonly occurs in the lumbosacral (L4/5 or L5/S1 discs) and lower cervical regions. A prolapsed L4/5 disc may produce pressure on the L4 exiting, or L5 traversing, nerves giving the patient symptoms corresponding to the affected myotome or dermatome.

Index